Breakfast Cookbook for Beginners

*100 Easy & Delicious Breakfast
Ideas & Breakfast Recipes*

Jerryk luna

Table of Contents

Introduction

First and foremost, I want to give a huge thank you for purchasing my book, '*Breakfast Cookbook for Beginners: 100 Easy & Delicious Breakfast Ideas & Breakfast Recipes*'

I hope you are prepared to experience one of the most wonderful cooking in the world from the comfort of your own kitchen.

In this book you will learn about the 100 easy & delicious Breakfast Recipes from eight countries. I am collect the best breakfast recipes from Sweden, Russia, Peru Norway, Nigeria, American Muffins & Morocco. All recipe with necessary kitchen equipment.

A food that is rich in both its flavors and colors.

Combined with local vegetation and amazing local herbs and spices, with traditional procedure. Incorporating some of the oldest cooking techniques on the planet, it consists of the heartiest of stews, some of the richest seafood dishes in the world, and of course the most decadent of deserts.

It offers more than enough to get you and your family through the Delicious Breakfast Ideas & Breakfast Recipes – so what are you waiting for? Dive on in and get exploring!

Chapter 1: Swedish Breakfast Recipes

Filmjölk Loaf with Lingonberry

Serves: 2-4

Ingreients:

- 400 ml filmjölk (natural yogurt or buttermilk)
- 180 g plain flour
- 120 g whole meal flour
- 65 g hazelnuts (coarsely chopped)
- 60 g lingonberries (fresh or frozen)
- 50 g spelt flakes
- 40 g rolled oats
- 4 teaspoon baking powder
- 1 loaf
- 1 teaspoon salt
- 1–2 tablespoons pumpkin seeds (for decoration)

Method:

1. First, preheat the oven to 200° C. Place oven paper in a bread tin that holds about 1½ liters.
2. Mix all the dry ingredients.
3. Add the filmjölk and mix together. Fold in the lingonberries and nuts.
4. Pour the mixer hooked on the tin and top with pumpkin seeds.
5. Bake for about 50 minutes. Consent to cool on wire holders, under a dry goods.

Jule Kaka (Swedish Christmas Bread with Candied fruits and Cardamom Flavor)

Serves: 6-8

Ingredients:

- 8 ½ cups all-purpose flour
- 2 (.25 ounce) packages active dry yeast
- 2 teaspoons salt
- 2 cups scalded milk
- 1 cup butter (melted)
- 1 cup golden raisins
- 1 medium egg white (beaten)
- 1 cup white sugar
- 1 tablespoon ground cardamom
- ½ cup warm water (110 F/45 C)
- ½ cup candied cherries (sliced)
- ½ cup candied citron (chopped)

Method:

1. Dissolve the yeast in water.
2. Scald milk, and add melted butter or margarine, salt, sugar. When lukewarm, add to yeast and water. Stir in 4 cups flour. Cover, and place in a warm place. Let it rise for about 2 hours, or until doubled in bulk.
3. Punch down. Stir in cardamom, cherries, raisins and citron. Work in remaining flour until soft dough forms. Let rise in warm place for 2 to 3 hours, or until doubled.
4. Knead slightly, and form into 4 round loaves. Place on greased cookie sheets. Let rise for 50 min to 100 min, or till doubled. Brush loaves with beaten egg white.

5. Bake at 350 degrees F (175 degrees C) for 30 to 40 minutes, or until golden brown.

Breakfast Rolls with Sour Cherry and Vanilla Jam

Serves: 8

Ingredients:

- 700g strong white bread flour (plus extra for dusting and sprinkling)
- 70g whole meal flour
- 25g fresh yeast
- 1 tablespoon honey
- 1 teaspoon salt

For the jam:

- 400g fresh or frozen sour cherries (or black cherries), stoned
- 150g golden caster sugar
- 1 vanilla pod (halved lengthways)
- ½ lemon (juiced)

Method:

1. First, crumble the yeast into the honey, add 1 teaspoon salt, then mix until the yeast dissolves. Add 600ml lukewarm water and mix thoroughly. Add the flours and mix into a sticky dough, but don't knead. Concealment the container with a tea cloth and consent to rise for about one hour.
2. In the meantime, make the jam. Put a saucer in the freezer. Combine the cherries, lemon juice and vanilla

pod in a small saucepot with 1 tablespoon sugar. Bring to a gentle simmer and stir until the sugar dissolves. Add another spoonful of sugar and repeat, continuing until it has all been added. Simmer for 20–30 minutes, or until jammy. Take the saucer from the freezer. Place 1 teaspoon of the jam on to it and leave for 1 minute or so to cool completely. Push a finger across the jam. If it creases, the jam is ready or else, cook it for a bit lengthier. Once complete, pour into a sterilized jar.

3. Set the oven to 220C/425F/gas 7 and lightly grease 2 baking sheets. Flatten the dough on a floured work surface – sprinkle with plenty of flour to make it easier to handle. Divide the dough into 8 pieces. Shape into about 8-10cm rounds. Transference on to the prepared baking sheets, spacing out evenly.

4. Sprinkling over a slightly extra flour, then bake for 16–18 minutes, or until golden.

5. Allow to cool a slightly before getting stuck in, slathering with jam.

Swedish Breakfast Buns

Serves: 4

Ingredients:

- 2 medium-large eggs
- 2 tablespoons psyllium husk powder
- 2 tablespoons olive oil (extra virgin, or light)
- 1 tablespoon whole flax seeds
- 1 tablespoon sunflower seeds (shelled)
- 1 teaspoon baking powder
- ¾ cup almond flour
- ½ teaspoon salt
- ½ cup sour cream (or creme fraiche)

Method:

1. Start by preheating the oven to 400 degrees.
2. Mix almond flour, seeds, psyllium, salt, and baking powder in a container.
3. Add eggs, olive oil, and sour cream and mix it carefully.
4. Let it sit for 5 minutes.
5. Cut the dough into 4 pieces. Shape into balls and put in a cake pot (We use a 9-inch circular pot, but anything really will work here so long as it has sides).
6. Use parchment paper to prevent sticking.
7. Bake for approximately 20-25 minutes until browned.

Risgrynsgröt (Swedish Rice Porridge)

Serves: 5-6

Ingredients:

- 4 ½ cups milk
- 1 ½ cups water
- 1 cup short-grained, glutinous rice (we use Jasmine because of its added sweetness; pearl rice also works well)
- 1 tablespoon butter
- ½ teaspoon salt
- cinnamon-sugar and butter to taste

Method:

1. First, rinse the rice well and drain.
2. In a heavy-bottomed saucepot, bring 1 ½ cups water, butter, and salt to a rapid boil over high heat.
3. Dispense in the rice, stirring continually to prevent stabbing.
4. Reduce the heat to low, stirring the rice until boiling is reduced to a simmer.
5. Cover the pot and simmer for 10 to 15 minutes, until the rice has absorbed most of the water.
6. Add the milk to the rice, stirring to incorporate. Bring the combination to a boil, stirring constantly, then immediately reduce the heat to low.
7. Once boiling has reduced to a simmer, cover the pot and allow it to cook, without stirring, for 45 minutes. Be careful here to avoid it scorching.
8. Serve warm with cinnamon-sugar and butter to taste.

Raggmunkar (Swedish Potato Potcake)

Serves: 4

Ingredients:

- 1 ½ lbs. Idaho or other baking potatoes
- 6-8 tablespoons clarified butter
- 1 Spotish onion (finely chopped)
- 1 large egg (lightly beaten)
- kosher salt and freshly ground black pepper

Method:

1. Start by preheating the oven to 300 F.
2. Peel the potatoes and superbly grate them on a box grater or the rough disk of a food processor. Wrap in a kitchen towel and turn it tightly to squeeze out as much liquid as probable. Put the potatoes in a large container and add the onion and egg, socializing well. Period with salt and pepper. Divide the potato combination into 3 parts.
3. Heat 1 ½ to 2 tablespoons of the clarified butter in an 8-inch skillet over medium heat (if you have two 8-inch skillets, cook 2 potcakes at a time). Add one quarter of the potato combination, pressing it into a flat cake with a spatula, and cook for 12 minutes, or until golden brown on the bottom.
4. Turn the cake and cook for about 10 minutes longer, or until browned on the bottom side and cooked through. Transference to paper towels to gutter briefly, then Transferenceence to a baking sheet and keep warm in the oven while you cook the remaining potcakes.
5. Serve hot.

Traditional Swedish Potcakes

Serves: 4

Ingredients:

- 3 medium-large eggs
- 2 ½ cups low-fat milk
- 1 ¼ cups flour
- ½ teaspoon salt
- three tablespoons butter or three tablespoons margarine (melted)

Method:

1. In a large mixing container, beat the eggs with 1/2 the milk.
2. Tired in flour and salt until smooth.
3. Stir in liquid butter and remaining milk.
4. Warmth a griddle or large skillet with a small amount of coconut oil.
5. For each potcake, pour about 1/4 cup batter onto the griddle and cook over medium heat 1 to 2 minutes.
6. With a spatula, chance the potcakes and cook until golden brown, about 1 minute.
7. Serve closely or keep warm while making the remaining potcakes.

Swedish (Egg) Coffee

Serves: 1

Ingredients:

- 8 cup filtered cool water
- 1 cup ground coffee of your choice
- 1 medium egg with the shell
- additional 1/3 cup water

Method:

1. Bring your 8 cups of water to a boil in a large pot. While your water is heating up, combine the coffee grounds, egg with the shell (give your shell a good washing beforehand), and 1/3 cup water in a separate container.
2. Allow the egg combination to rest while the water comes to a boil.
3. Once it's boiling, add in the coffee-omelet combination. Once you do, it will foam a bit, this is normal.
4. As soon as it comes back to a boil, turn off the heat and remove it from the stove. Allow it to set for 6-7 minutes, or longer if you like it really strong. The hot water cooks the eggs, so the coffee grounds will clump together and float in chunks.
5. After 6-7 minutes, slowly pour the coffee through a fine mesh strainer.
6. Add cream and taste it before you add any sweetener.

Kanelbullar (Swedish Cinnamon Butterhorns)

Serves: 4

Ingredients:

- 6 cups all-purpose flour
- 3 medium-large eggs
- 1 package (¾ oz or 21 g) active dry yeast
- 1 ½ cup milk
- ½ cup unsalted butter
- ½ cup sugar
- ½ teaspoon salt
- ¼ cup warm water (ideally between 90-115 F)

Filling:

- 1 tablespoon cinnamon
- ¾ cup sugar
- ½ cup softened butter

Egg wash:

- 1 medium-large egg beaten with 2 tablespoons milk

Method:

1. In a small saucepot over medium heat, warm milk until hot, then add butter and stir until butter is dissolved. Remove from heat and set aside. In a small dish, add yeast to warm water and let stand for 4 minutes. Temporarily, beat together eggs, sugar, and salt in a large container, then beat in cooled milk as well as yeast combination. Add flour in two additions, mixing well to

make a plane but thick batter. Cover and refrigerate at least 3 and up to 23 hours.

2. When you are ready to bake, preheat oven to 375 F and line a baking sheet with parchment or a silicone baking liner. Remove dough from the fridge and divide into three parts. Working with one ¼ of the dough, roll it into a ball using your hands, then Transference it to a well-floured surface and roll it into a 12-inch circle. Spread ¼ of the softened butter on the dough round, then mix together sugar and cinnamon and sprinkle ¼ of the combination over the butter.

3. Using a sharp knife or pizza cutter, slice the round into 8 wedges. Starting at the wide, outer edge of one of the wedges, roll the dough towards the inside, pointed edge, forming a crescent shaped roll. Transferenceence to the lined baking sheet and repeat with the remaining dough. Cover the rolls with a towel and let rise for about 45 minutes in a draft-free area.

4. Before baking, lightly brush the tops of the rolls with the egg wash, and sprinkle with a bit of sugar. Bake at 380 degrees for 11-14 minutes, until golden brown on the tops. Cool on baking sheet on a cooling rack, then Transferenceence Kanelbullar to an airtight container. Will keep for 2-3 days, or longer if refrigerated and well-sealed.

5. A few teaspoons of granulated sugar for sprinkling on the top. Can be served warm or at room temperature.

Gluten Free Swedish Potcakes

Serves: 3-4

Ingredients:

- 3 medium-large eggs (room temperature)
- 2 teaspoons pure vanilla extract
- 1 tablespoon granulated sugar
- 1 ½ cups milk of choice (but not canned coconut milk as it's too thick)
- ¼ teaspoon salt
- ¾ cup + 2 tablespoons certified gluten free oat flour
- butter (for frying)

Method:

1. Use an immersion blender or a blender to blend all the ingredients together until thoroughly combined and no lumps remain. You can also mix it by hand and make sure to stir the batter very well before pouring the batter into the pot.
2. Heat a 9″ skillet over medium heat and melt about 1 teaspoon of butter in the pot. Tilt the pot to cover the whole pot in butter. Pour 1/4 cup of batter into the pot. Very quickly tilt the pot to swirl the batter evenly all around the pot. Cook for about two minute or until the bottom is golden brown and then carefully flip it over and cook for about another 35 seconds or until cooked.
3. Serve immediately with fruit sauce, jam, or preserves.

Swedish Tea Ring

Serves: 2 rings (48 servings)

Ingredients:

- 8 to 9 cups flour
- 1-quart whole milk
- 1 cup butter
- 1 cup sugar
- 2 teaspoons baking powder
- 1 ½ tablespoons yeast

For the filling:

- 2 to 3 cups butter (melted)
- 2 cups sugar
- 1 cup golden raisins
- 1 cup raisins
- 1 cup pecans (chopped)
- ¼ cup cinnamon

For the icing:

- 4 cups powdered sugar
- 1 teaspoon almond extract
- ½ teaspoon vanilla extract
- 1/8 cup whole milk

Method:

1. First, heat the milk, butter, and sugar in a saucepot over medium heat, getting it to a simmer, but not a boil. Remove from the heat and let it cool to lukewarm. This

may take 10 minutes or so. You can transference it to the fridge in another container if you need to speed up the process.

2. Pour the yeast over the top of the milk combination and stir to combine. Then, add 7 cups of the flour and stir together gently. Cover with a towel and put it in a warm place to rise for about 1 hour.
3. Add the rest of the flour and the baking powder and stir to combine.
4. Divide the dough into two or three large pieces.
5. Roll out one piece at a time into a large rectangle. Leave it relatively thick, about ½ inch. Make sure the rectangle is long, width-wise. (Think hot dog, not hamburger.)
6. Pour about ¾ cup of butter over the dough and sprinkle about half the cinnamon and sugar over the top.
7. Top with half of the dried fruits and chopped pecans.
8. Roll the dough away from you in a tight roll until it is completely rolled up. Pinch the seam together and then cut into 3-inch slices.
9. Bring the two ends of the roll together and pinch them together. Gently Transference onto a parchment lined baking sheet.
10. Cut large slits ¾ of the way through the dough, make about 10 cuts. Turn each cut section onto its side.
11. Brush the top of the ring with melted butter and cover gently with a cloth. Repeat with the rest of the dough. Let it rise for about 30 minutes. While it is rising, preheat the oven to 375 F.
12. Bake rolls for about 25 minutes, do not over bake. They should be lightly brown and slightly firm to the touch. Tent with some foil if it is frying too quickly.
13. Whisk together the powdered sugar, milk, almond extract, and vanilla extract. If it is too thick add a slightly

more milk, if it is too thin add a slightly more powdered sugar.

14. Remove rings from the oven and if you can manage let them cool a bit and then drizzle icing over the top, slice and serve!

Kroppkakor (Potato Dumplings Stuffed with Bacon and Onion)

Serves: 14 dumplings

Ingredients:

- 3 lb. russet potatoes (peeled and cut into 1" pieces)
- 1 lb. sliced bacon (roughly chopped)
- 2 ½ cups flour (plus more for dusting)
- 2 medium eggs (plus 1 yolk)
- 1 large yellow onion (minced)
- 1 tablespoon olive oil
- 1 tablespoon ground allspice
- lingonberry preserves and sour cream (for serving)
- salt to taste

Method:

1. Start with boiling the potatoes in a 4-qt. saucepot of salted water until tender, about 20 minutes. Drain potatoes and let cool, then Transference to a container and mash until smooth. Add some flour, eggs, yolk, and salt; stir to combine. Cover with plastic wrap and chill dough 35 minutes.

2. Heat oil and bacon in a 12" skillet over medium-high heat; cook until fat is just rendered, 10–12 minutes. Add some onion and cook, stirring occasionally, until onion is golden and bacon is crisp, about 7 minutes. Decant off and discard fat, or save for another use. Stirring allspice and salt into bacon combination; let cool.

3. Bring an 8-qt. saucepot of salted water to a boil. On a informally floured surface, divide dough into fourteen 5-

oz. balls. Working with 1 ball dough at a time and with lightly dusted hands, press index finger into center of ball to create a pocket; place about 2 tbsp. bacon combination inside pocket and pinch edges of dough to seal; roll into a smooth ball and flatten into a 2 1/2"-wide patty about 1" thick. Add dumplings to water; when dumplings float, reduce the heat to medium and simmer until firm, about 30 minutes. Using a slotted spoon, Transference the dumplings to a serving platter.

4. Serve with lingonberry preserves and sour cream.

Chapter 2: Russian Breakfast recipes

Blini (potcakes)

Makes: 40

Ingredients

- 5 cups milk

- 1 cup all-purpose flour

- 2 tablespoons white sugar

- 2 tablespoons butter

- 4 eggs

- 2 tablespoon vegetable oil

- 2/3 teaspoon salt

Method

1. Take a medium container and whisk in – the eggs, salt, and sugar. Carefully, sift the flour in with the milk. Mix until everything is properly combined. The batter needs to be thin in consistency.

2. Heat a skillet or griddle – make sure it's on medium heat. Use cooking spray or lightly oil the pot to grease it.

3. Using a big spoon or a ladle, pour around 2 tablespoons of batter, or however much you require, in the pot. Tilt the pot around so that the batter spreads out evenly.

4. Once the edges start looking a bit crisp and the middle looks dry, carefully slide a spatula under the blini and flip it. Cook the other side for about a minute, or until it has browned a bit.

5. Transference the blini to a plate. Top it with some butter then keep stacking the blini on top of one another.

6. When serving, serve with a filling of your choice. Place the filling in the middle; fold the blini in half, then half again, so it forms a triangle.

Zapekanka (Farmer's cheese breakfast cake)

Makes: 2 loaves (9 x 5inches each)

Ingredients

- 1 cup organic cane sugar

- 1 cup sea salt or kosher salt

- Zest of 2 large lemon or oranges

- 4 tablespoons of semolina (Farina, Cream of Wheat)

- 8 extra large eggs at room temperature

- 5 cups well drained ricotta cheese

- 1 cup sour cream combined with 1 teaspoon each of – lemon juice and baking soda

- 4 teaspoons of pure vanilla extract

- 1/2 cup of each – mini chocolate chips, chopped candied orange or any other citrus peel, and chopped dried fruit or berries that have been soaked in brandy or rum.

Method

1. Preheat the oven to 325 F.

2. Take two 9 x 5 inches loaf tins and butter them. Then line the bottoms using parchment then butter the parchment paper lightly as well. This ensures easy de-molding of the cake.

3. In a large mixing container, beat the sugar with the eggs together until the combination turns light and kind of fluffy and the color is a pale yellow. It will take around 8-10 minutes to achieve this.

4. In another container, whisk the cheese, sour cream combination, vanilla and orange (or lemon) zest until everything is properly combined and smooth.

5. Slowly and carefully add the egg combination and sugar until everything is nicely incorporated. Then add the semolina.

6. Use a spatula to slowly fold in the mini chocolate chips, the soaked and drained fruit and berries, and the candied citrus peel.

7. Allow the batter to rest for at least 20-30 minutes. This lets the semolina to swell and helps in absorbing the excess moisture present in the batter.

8. Pour this batter into loaf tins you have prepared use a spatula to even out the surface of the batter.

9. Place them on the center rack of the oven. Bake for around 40-50 minutes until the cakes have turned golden brown and the center does not jiggle.

10. Once they are done, place the tins on a wire rack to let the cakes cool in the molds for around 20 minutes. Take a paring knife and run it around the edges, and invert the cakes on to a serving platter.

Draniki (savory potato potcakes)

Makes: 8

Ingredients

For the batter:

- 20 ounces of potatoes

- 2 tablespoons of flour

- 2 egg yolks

- Salt to taste

- Pepper to taste

For the filling:

- 20 ounces of ground pork

- 2 clove of garlic, minced

- 1/2 teaspoon cumin powder

- 1/3 onion, minced

- Pepper to taste

- Salt to taste

For the cucumber sauce:

- 2 cucumbers, grated

- 2 teaspoons fresh dill, chopped

- 6 tablespoons mayonnaise

- 2 tablespoons lemon juice

- Pepper to taste

- Salt to taste

Method:

1. Wash, peel, and then grate the potatoes. You can even opt for a food processor to blend until it is smooth. Use a sieve to drain out the excess water. Then add the rest of the batter ingredients and mix until well incorporated.

2. In a separate container, mix all the ingredients of the filling, and divide it into four and set it aside.

3. For the sauce, mix all the ingredients listed for it in a small container.

4. Heat a frying pot with a bit of oil. Ladle around four spoonfuls of potato combination separately on to the pot. Make sure the mounds are at least an inch away from each other. Top each mound with a portion of the pork filling, and then follow it with another spoonful of potato combination to cover the top, do this for each mound.

5. Cook on both sides until they are nice and brown. Serve hot with the cucumber sauce you have prepared.

Kasha

Makes: 8 servings

Ingredients

- 1/2 cup buckwheat groats

- 1 tablespoon sugar

- 1/2 teaspoon salt

- 1 ¾ cups of milk

- 1 ounce of butter

Method

1. Take the groats and cleanse them. And to cleanse them you need to put them in a small to medium pot – pour cold water over the groats then simply stir the groats with a whisk then drain out the dirty water. Add some more water, whisk it again and drain one last time.

2. Add 2 cups of water to the cleansed groats, add salt then cook until all the water boils over.

3. Add the milk, butter, and sugar to the buckwheat. Bring it to a boil and once it starts boiling - remove it from the heat.

4. Pour into containers and enjoy this slightly sweet variation of the regular kasha.

Grenki (sweet toasts)

Makes: 16

Ingredients

- 8 slices of bread (opt for a sweet variety of bread to yield better results)

- 2 tablespoons of granulated sugar

- 1 cup heavy cream

- ¼ teaspoon ground cinnamon

- 4 large eggs

- ¼ teaspoon salt

- 4 tablespoons oil

- ½ cup milk

Method

1. Slicing them diagonally cut the slices of bread in half.

2. In a container, whisk in the egg, milk, salt, cinnamon, sugar, and cream, until everything is properly combined.

3. Heat some oil in a griddle or skillet.

4. Coat each piece of bread by dipping it into the egg combination then placing it on the medium hot pot.

5. Cook each side until the color is golden brown.

Syrniki (cottage cheese potcakes)

Makes: 8 servings

Ingredients

- 2 cup cottage cheese

- 6 tablespoons all-purpose flour, plus more for dusting

- 6 tablespoons white sugar

- 4 tablespoons semolina

- 4 eggs, beaten

- 4-6 tablespoons canola oil

Method

1. In a container mix in the cottage cheese, sugar, and eggs until everything is well combined.

2. Stir in the all-purpose flour and semolina, and carefully work the combination into a soft dough.

3. Flour your working surface, place the dough, sprinkle some more flour on it and divide it into 8 equal pieces. Lightly pat down each piece to form patties that are at least half inch in thickness.

4. Take the oil in a pot and place it over medium heat. Once hot, place as many syrniki as would fit in your pot, leaving ample space for you to turn them without breaking the neighboring ones. Flip the syrniki after the bottom has cooked to a light brown shade, and cook on

the other side until you notice the same. It generally takes 3-4 minutes on either side.

Guryevskaya – semolina porridge

Makes – 5-6

Ingredients

- 34 fl ounces of milk

- 1 ½ cups of sugar or vanilla sugar

- 2 cups of semolina

- 3 cups of berries – fresh or frozen

- ½ cup of almonds

- 4-5 tablespoons of butter

- 4 eggs

For the syrup –

- ½ cup of berries, crushed – fresh or frozen

- 2 tablespoons of sugar

- Cinnamon powder

Method Syrup –

1. In a small saucepot, add in the crushed berries and place it over low-medium heat.

2. Add in the sugar and a pinch ground cinnamon powder. Keep stirring everything.

3. Let the syrup come to a boil.

4. Once it starts boiling, reduce the heat and allow the syrup to simmer for around 3-4 minutes.

5. Once done, Transference the syrup to a container and set it aside until it is time for it to be used.

Porridge –

1. Take a saucepot and add in the milk and sugar. Set the heat to medium and bring it to a boil. Once it starts boiling, proceed to the next step.

2. Carefully and gradually start adding in the semolina.

3. Keep stirring and allow it to boil for about 10 minutes. Make sure you keep stirring so that there are no lumps forming.

4. Remove the saucepot from the heat then add in the raw eggs and the butter and keep mixing it.

5. Once everything comes together properly, take the almond in a blender pot or a food processor and mill them until they have turned into a powder.

6. Prepare a casserole or a baking ban by greasing it with some butter. Make sure you grease the corners well.

7. Add in half or more of the almond powder to the casserole or baking pot that you have prepared and make sure you even out the almond powder properly.

8. Next, place the berries by laying them out and spreading them over the almond layer evenly.

9. Carefully pour the porridge that you have boiled and spread it out evenly then sprinkle the top with some more sugar and what is remaining of the almond powder.

10. Pop the prepared porridge into a preheated oven at 350F for 10 to 15 minutes.

11. Once done, pour the syrup over the porridge and add in some more berries to decorate it.

12. Serve hot and enjoy!

Vareniki

Makes – 2-3 servings

Ingredients

For the dough –

- 1 cup of all purpose flour – unbleached
- 1 large egg yolk
- 4 tablespoons of water
- 2 tablespoons of unsalted butter
- ½ tablespoon of vegetable oil
- Salt – as per taste
- 1 egg white, beaten lightly

For the filling –

- 2 cups of sour cherries, freshly pitted or use jarred
- ½ tablespoon of cornstarch
- ¼ cup of sugar if using fresh cherries and 2-3 tablespoons of sugar if using jarred cherries
- 3 tablespoons of cherry flavored liqueur
- 3 tablespoons of unsalted butter
- Cherry juice, as required

Method

For the cherry filling –

1. If using jarred cherries, make sure you drain the cherries thoroughly and also reserve at least a cup of that syrup instead of throwing it away. In a small container mix the sugar and the jarred cherries. Keep a few cherries aside to be used for garnishing.

2. If using fresh berries – in a small container mix the cherries with the sugar and leave the container somewhere warm for a few hours or until they start giving off their juices. Strain out the juice – you should be left with about a cup of the cherry juice. And if you have less than a cup then add some bottled or canned cherry juice to compensate for it.

3. Take a saucepot that is small in size then add in the juice or syrup that you have reserved. Place the saucepot over medium to high heat then bring it to a boil. Allow it to boil until the juice or syrup has reduced to half of its initial quantity.

4. Take the saucepot off the heat then add in the liqueur and keep stirring as you add it in. Set it aside and allow it to cool. You are going to use this to pour it over the cooked vareniki.

5. As for the cherries – add them to a container along with the cornstarch and toss both of them together. Set aside until it's time to use the filling.

Dough, assembling, and cooking –

1. Blend the salt and flour using a food processor. And while the motor is still running, add in the oil and egg yolk through the processor's feed tube.

2. Next, pour the water in but make sure you are pouring it in a slow and steady stream until the combination starts forming into a ball around the processor's blades and resembles a ball of dough.

3. Lightly flour a working surface and Transference the dough to it. Knead the dough until it is smooth − it will take around 2 minutes to achieve that. Cover the dough with a damp cloth and let it rest for around 30 minutes.

4. Roll the dough out on a floured surface using a rolling pin that has also been floured lightly. You need to roll the dough out into a really thin sheet that is about 1/16" in thickness, and ensure the sheet is not tearing anywhere!

5. Use a round cookie cutter or a glass and start cutting out circles that are around 3" in diameter. Whatever scraps remain − instead of throwing them away, simply gather and knead them into a small dough and place a damp cloth over them. You are going to make your last batch of vareniki using that.

6. Beat an egg white in a small container and keep it within reach.

7. Place about a heaping teaspoon of the cherry filling in the center of each circle of the dough. While measuring the teaspoon of filling, use 2-3 cherries if fresh, 4 if you've used canned cherries)

8. Carefully fold the vareniki dough over your cherry filling and form a semi circle. Brush the dough's edges with the

beaten egg white then press those edges down firmly together using a fork. This will help seal the filling in. as you are shaping the vareniki, place each shaped one on a large baking tray that has been floured lightly. Make sure you are placing them an inch apart from each other. Cover the shaped vareniki with a damp cloth.

9. Use the remaining piece of dough compiled from the scrap and shape as many vareniki as you can out of it.

10. Add 10 cups of salted water to a large pot and bring it to a boil. Once it starts boiling, bring the heat down to medium to let the water simmer then carefully add the vareniki to the simmering water. Instead of just dropping the vareniki, lower them into the water gently.

11. Boil and stir occasionally using a wooden spoon to prevent the vareniki from sticking to each other. Boil until the vareniki start rising to the surface and have cooked through. It will take about 6-7 minutes.

12. Once done, carefully take them out of the water using a slotted spoon and place them in a colander. Drain the vareniki as thoroughly as you can.

13. Transference them to a serving container and toss them with the butter.

14. Serve with the reserved and concentrated cherry syrup drizzled on top.

Savory Nalesniki

Makes – 3 servings (6 crepes)

Ingredients

For the crepes –

- ¼ cup lukewarm water

- 2 large eggs

- ½ cup of milk

- 2 tablespoons plus more of unsalted butter, melted

- 1/8 teaspoon of salt

- ½ cup of all purpose flour

For the filling –

- 4 ounces of leftover turkey meat – white and/or dark meat

- 4 ounces of mushrooms, sliced

- 1 ½ tablespoon of olive oil

- ½ of a medium sized onion, chopped finely

- ½-1 tablespoon of water

- ½ tablespoon of olive oil

- ½ carrot – grated finely

- ¼ teaspoon of salt and a dash of pepper

Method Crepes –

1. Add all of the crepe ingredients to the blender and combine them. Blend until you get a smooth and lump free batter.

2. Melt a bit of butter in a medium sized skillet on medium heat. Pour around 2-3 tablespoons of the batter in the skillet and instantly swirl the skillet to let the batter spread and coat the pot's bottom. If there are any cracks or holes, fill in with a bit of batter.

3. Do not potic if the first crepe is not the most aesthetic one.

4. Once the bottom side of the crepe has turned a light golden in color, flip it using a spatula with a thin edge. It might take around less than a minute, but that depends on how hot your pot in.

5. Repeat with the rest of the batter and let your crepes cool down on a chopping board for a couple of minutes then stack them up.

For the filling –

1. Place a skillet on medium-high heat. Add in 1 ½ tablespoon of olive oil. Add in the sliced mushrooms, finely chopped onions, and finely grated carrot. Sauté them all until they are soft and keep stirring everything occasionally. It will take around 7 to 10 minutes for them to soften up. Season with pepper and salt.

2. Using a meat grinder that has a big holed attachment – grind the turkey up along with the onion, carrot, and mushroom combination. Stir everything and make sure the ingredients are properly combined. Add ½ tablespoon of olive oil followed by about a tablespoon of water.

3. Take the turkey combination and spread about 2 tablespoons of it over each crepe. Spread the combination out up to the edges using a spatula.

4. You can fold the crepes in half twice to make triangular crepes or simply roll them like logs.

5. Serve with dollops of sour cream.

Chapter 3: Peruvian Breakfast Recipes

Tacu Tacu (Beans and Rice)

Serves: 4

Ingredients

- 400 g tin of haricot beans
- 300 g long-grain white rice
- 4 medium-large free-range eggs
- 2 cloves of garlic
- 1 plantain
- 1 onion
- 1 fresh red chili
- olive oil
- hot chili sauce

Method

1. Start by cooking the rice according to packet instructions, then drain and cool.
2. Peel and slice the plantain about 1.5cm thick. Peel and finely chop the garlic and onion, then finely slice the chili. Drain the beans.
3. Add a couple of good lugs of oil to a large non-stick frying pot over a medium heat and fry the plantain for a few minutes on each side, or until golden and crisp. Set aside and keep warm.
4. Return the pot, with any leftover oil, to the heat. Fry the garlic, onion and chili over a medium-low heat for 5 to 10 minutes, or until softened and lightly golden.
5. Stir in 1 tablespoon of hot chili sauce, the beans and cooled rice.
6. Turn the heat up to high and fry the combination until the rice is piping hot and beginning to crisp up, stirring

regularly. Stop stirring for the last couple of minutes to let it get golden and crisp on the bottom – this is your tacu tacu! Transference to a plate and set aside.

7. Add a slightly more oil to the same pot and place over a medium heat. Fry the eggs, with the plantain for the last minute to warm through.

8. Split among your plates, making sure everybody gets some of that lovely crispy bottom, and top each portion with a fried egg, some crispy plantain and an additional dash of chili mush, if you like.

Potatoes in a Spicy Cheese Sauce

Serves: 8

Ingredients

- 14 ounces queso blanco (fresh white cheese)
- 8 yukon gold potatoes
- 6 medium-large black olives (halved)
- 4 leaves lettuce (or more to taste)
- 4 yellow chili peppers
- 2 garlic cloves
- 2 medium-large hard-boiled eggs (halved)
- 1 teaspoon olive oil
- ½ cup vegetable oil
- 2 tablespoons heavy whipping cream, or more as needed (optional)

Method

1. First, bring a large pot of water to a boil. Add the potatoes; cook until tender when pierced with a fork, about 30-45 minutes. Drain and let cool, about 15 minutes.
2. Heat olive oil in a small saucepot. Add yellow chili peppers and garlic cloves; cook and stir until lightly golden, about 2 minutes.
3. Transference chili peppers and garlic cloves to a blender. Add queso blanco and vegetable oil; blend until smooth. Thin with heavy cream until a creamy constancy is reached.
4. Arrange lettuce leaves on a large platter. Cut potatoes in half and place on top. Pour sauce over potatoes.

5. Garnish with hard-boiled eggs and black olives.

Chicharrones Sandwich with Salsa Criolla

Serves: 2-4

Ingredients

Chicharrones de chancho (crispy pork cubes):

- 1 lb. pork spare ribs (cut into 2-inch sections)
- 1 teaspoon salt
- 1 tablespoon lime juice
- 1 teaspoon oil
- ½ teaspoon ground cumin

Salsa criolla:

- 3-4 tablespoons lime juice
- 2 cups red onion (coarsely chopped)
- 1 teaspoon chopped/paste aji amarillo, remove seeds if chopping.
- 1 teaspoon salt
- 1 tablespoon cilantro (chopped)

Method

For the Chicharrones de chancho (crispy pork cubes):

1. First, mix all ingredients except oil in a container and let marinate for 15 minutes.
2. Heat oil in a skillet or a pot on low heat.
3. Add the pork and fry at low temperatures for about 30 minutes.
4. The pork is done when the meat is brown and crisp with all of the fat cooked off.

5. Drain pieces over paper towels and serve as soon as possible.

For the salsa criolla:

1. Combine all ingredients by hand, or
2. Pulse all ingredients in a food processor to make a coarse salsa.
3. Serve immediately.

Ceviche Peruano

Serves: 8

Ingredients

- 1-pound fresh tilapia (cut into 1/2-inch pieces)
- 1.5-pound medium shrimp (peeled, deveined, and cut into 2-inch pieces)
- 2 medium-large potatoes
- 2 medium sweet potatoes
- 1 red onion (cut into thin strips)
- 1 cup fresh lime juice
- 1 pinch ground cumin
- 1 clove garlic (minced)
- 1 habanero pepper (seeded and minced)
- 1 bibb or Boston lettuce (separated into leaves)
- ½ stalk celery (sliced)
- ¼ cup lightly packed cilantro leaves
- salt and pepper to taste

Method

6. Start with placing the potatoes and sweet potatoes in a saucepot and cover with water. Boil until the potatoes are easily stabbed with a fork, then drain, and set aside to cool to normal temperature.
7. Place the sliced onion in a container of warm water, let stand 10 minutes, then drain and set aside.
8. In the meantime, place the lime juice, celery, cilantro, and cumin into the container of a blender, and puree until smooth. Pour this combination into a large glass container, and stir in the garlic and habanero pepper.

9. Season with salt and pepper, then stir in the diced tilapia and shrimp.
10. Set aside to marinate for an hour, stirring occasionally. The seafood is complete once it turns firm and milky.
11. To serve, peel the potatoes and cut into slices. Stir the onions into the fish combination. Line serving containers with lettuce leaves. Spoon the ceviche with its juice into the containers and garnish with slices of potato.

Peruvian Causa (Spicy Potato-Layered with Meat)

Serves: 8

Ingredients

- 8 medium russet potatoes (peeled)
- 3 hard-boiled eggs (thinly sliced)
- 2 (5 ounce) cans tuna (drained)
- 2 medium avocados (cut into thin strips)
- 2 tablespoons aji amarillo (minced)
- 1 small red onion (diced small)
- ½ cup vegetable oil (or as needed)
- ½ cup mayonnaise (divided)
- salt and pepper to taste

Method

6. First, place the potatoes into a large pot and cover with salted water; bring to a boil. Reduce heat to medium-low and boil until fond, about 25 minutes. Drain.
7. Mash potatoes with a ricer or hand mixer until smooth. Slowly stir in oil until potatoes come together; add aji amarillo, salt, and pepper.
8. Cool potato combination in the refrigerator, about 20 minutes.
9. Stir tuna, onion, and ¼ cup mayonnaise together in a container.
10. Line a casserole dish with plastic wrap. Spread ½ the potato combination on the bottom of the dish. Spread 2 tablespoons mayonnaise over the potatoes, spread the tuna combination over the mayonnaise, and place the

avocado slices in a single layer on top of the tuna combination.

11. Spread the remaining ½ of potato combination over the avocados, and top with remaining 2 tablespoons mayonnaise. Place sliced eggs over the top. Cover casserole dish with soft wrap and refrigerate until firm, about 35 minutes.

12. Invert casserole dish onto a serving dish or baking sheet to remove potato casserole from dish.

13. Remove plastic wrap and cut casserole into squares.

Desayuno Lurín

Serves: 4

Ingredients

For the pork belly:

- 4 lb. pork meat (preferably ribs)
- ½ lb. onion (julienned)
- salt to taste

For the tamales:

- 1 lb. chicken (shredded)
- 10 onion (chopped)
- 10 corn cobs (grated)
- ½ lb. lard
- 1/8 lb. toasted peanuts
- 12 black olives (pits removed)
- 4 mirasol peppers (deveined and seeds removed)
- 3 medium eggs (boiled)
- 3 garlic cloves
- plantain leaves (washed)
- salsa criolla, to taste
- salt and pepper, to taste

Method

For the pork belly:

1. In a pot of water, boil the pork meat until all the water evaporates and the meat begins to brown with its own fat. Once the meat has fried in its own fat and it looks browned, drain the excess fat.

1. Serve immediately with a side of fried sweet potato.

For the tamales:

1. Cook the grated corn in a pot of water for 5 minutes. Drain the water. Process the corn with a slightly vegetable oil until it makes a paste.
2. In a frying pot add 2 tablespoons of lard, add corn paste and stir continuously. Add chicken and remaining ingredients, including chicken stock. Cook until the corn paste is fully prepared and has thickened.
3. Add a slightly of the cooked corn combination to a plantain leaf, a piece of chicken, ¼ of boiled egg, toasted corn and 3 olives. Cover it with some more of the corn combination. Fold the tamale and cover it with strips of plantain leaves.
4. Once you have the tamales ready, cook them in a large pot of water for 1 hour. Once ready serve them with salsa criolla.
5. Invert casserole dish onto a serving dish or baking sheet to remove potato casserole from dish.

Locro Ecuatoriano (Potato-Cheese Soup)

Serves: 4

Ingredients

- 1 ½ pounds potatoes (or more to taste, peeled and diced)
- 4 cups chicken stock
- 3 cloves garlic (or more to taste, minced)
- 1 cup milk
- 1 cup shredded Muenster cheese
- ½ onion (minced)
- ¼ cup butter
- salt and pepper to taste

Method

1. Start by melting the butter in a large pot over medium heat. Cook and stir onion and garlic in hot butter until onion is glowing, 6 to 8 minutes.
2. Stir potatoes, chicken stock, and milk with the onion combination; season with salt and pepper. Bring the liquid to a boil, reduce heat to low, and cook at a simmer until potatoes are tender and falling apart, 30 to 45 minutes.
3. Mash potatoes lightly to help thicken the soup, while keeping some chunks in the soup.
4. Remove pot from heat and stir cheese into the soup to melt.

Peruvian Quinoa Porridge

Serves: 4

Ingredients

- 2 tablespoons coconut sugar (or honey)
- 2 cups rice milk (or Brazil nut milk)
- 1 cup quinoa
- 1 cup amaranth
- 1 teaspoon cloves
- 1 teaspoon cinnamon
- 1 scoop vanilla protein
- 1 teaspoon sea salt

Method

1. First, heat the nut milk with cloves and cinnamon. Slowly add coconut sugar to it.
2. After boiling for about 15 minutes, strain out the ingredients, and allow the nut milk to cool.
3. Cook the quinoa and amaranth separately in a pot.
4. Once the grains are done, Transference as much as needed to the milk to reach desired consistency.
5. Using a ladle, you can stir the combination.
6. Add the vanilla protein at this point.
7. You can serve this warm or store it in the refrigerator and serve it cold.

Frijoles Escabechados

Serves: 5

Ingredients

- 4 slices bacon
- 2 cups dried black beans (such as turtle beans, or 3 cups canned)
- 1 chile pepper (aji Amarillo, or other fresh chile pepper, seeds removed, sliced thinly)
- 1 tablespoon minced garlic
- 1 tablespoon chili pepper (aji potca, paste)
- 1 teaspoon cumin
- 1 packet sazon goya (with cilantro and tomato)
- 1 large white onion
- ¼ rice wine vinegar
- salt and pepper to taste

Method

1. First, soak dried beans overnight.
2. Drain and cover with clean water, and bring to a simmer. Add a slice of bacon, and simmer beans until tender. Sewer, reserving about 1 cup of the cooking liquid.
3. Add remaining 3 pieces of bacon to a large skillet and fry until crispy. Remove from pot, crumble, and set aside.
4. Slice onions into thin half-moon shaped pieces ("a la pluma"). Add onion and garlic to the same skillet with the aji chile pepper paste, cumin, and the sazon Goya, and cook them in the bacon grease over medium heat until they are golden brown, soft, and translucent. Add the sliced chile pepper and sauté for several minutes more.

5. Puree half of the beans in a blender with the reserved cooking liquid. Add the pureed beans to the skillet and simmer, stirring, for several minutes.
6. Add the remaining beans, the vinegar, and the crumbled bacon. Cook, stirring until beans are heated through.
7. Serve warm with white rice.

Gachas De Estilo Peruano (Peruvian Style Porridge)

Serves: 6

Ingredients

Manjar blanco & potthers milk:

- 200 ml single cream
- 200 ml condensed milk
- 5 cm green chili (frozen & finely grated)
- 5 cm red chili (frozen & finely grated)
- 5 cm cinnamon stick
- 4 cloves
- 3 tablespoons pisco
- 3 tablespoons lime juice
- 1 teaspoon vanilla bean paste
- pinch sea salt
- a squeeze of mango juice

Spiced coconut porridge:

- 1500 ml rude health coconut drink
- 350 g rude health 5 grain 6 seed porridge
- 6 tablespoons coconut sugar
- 6 tablespoons desiccated coconut
- 3 tablespoons vanilla bean paste
- 1 tablespoon ground cinnamon
- pinch salt

Candied cashews, mango & sweet potato ceviche & mango crisps:

- 150 g granulated sugar (plus extra for dusting)
- 100 g cashew nuts
- 100 ml water
- 1 lime (zested)
- ¾ mango (brunoise)
- ¾ cooked sweet potato (brunoise)
- ¼ mango (thinly sliced)

Method

1. Combine ingredients for manjar blanco in a small pot the day before serving. Take to the boil and reduce the heat to low. Simmer, stirring often for 2-3 hours until thick and caramelized. Taste and adjust the spicing to your liking then leave to cool and refrigerate.

2. For the lime, place 100 g of sugar in a pot with water and bring to the boil.

3. Whilst this is heating, pour a kettle of water over the lime zest and soak for 30 seconds. Drain, refresh in cold water and repeat (this will remove any bitterness).

4. Boil the zest in the sugar syrup for 5 minutes, drain, sprinkle with sugar and leave to set on a rack. Once set, store in an airtight jar.

5. For the cashews, place the sugar in a wide pot over a medium heat to dissolve the sugar. Swirl the pot but do not stir. Once the sugar is bubbling, leave to turn amber in color and add the cashews. Swirl to coat and pour onto baking parchment. Leave to set and break up when cool. Store in an airtight jar.

6. Mix all the porridge ingredients in a large pot and soak for 10 minutes.

7. Place pot on a medium heat and allow to cook for 15-20 minutes until the oats are tender but maintain a bit of bite (top the oats up with water if they become too thick).
8. Meanwhile, mix the ingredients for the potthers milk in a container and use to marinade the ceviche ingredients for 10 minutes.
9. Once the porridge is ready, serve, topped with ceviche (draining off some of the potthers milk before serving), Manjar Blanco, candied cashews and lime zest, and mango crisps.

Huevos Tripados Peruvian Tomatoes and Egg Noodles

Serves: 6

Ingredients

Noodles

- 9 medium-large eggs
- 1 tablespoon clarified butter *(see note)*
- ½ teaspoon coarse sea salt
- ¼ teaspoon ground black pepper
- ½ cup grated Mexican Manchego cheese
- 1/8 cup water biscuits (finely crushed)

Tomato sauce:

- 9 plum tomatoes
- 3 tablespoons olive oil
- 2 teaspoons ground fennel seeds
- 2 large cloves garlic (minced)
- 1 medium onion (minced)
- 1 teaspoon paprika
- 1 teaspoon cayenne pepper
- 1 bay leaf
- 1 tablespoon coarse sea salt
- 1 small carrot (grated)
- ½ small bunch fresh basil (leaves only, coarsely chopped)

Method

1. Start by breaking the eggs one by one, into a small container, then slide them into a large mixing container. Add ½ cup cold water, the salt, and pepper. Whisk together until evenly mixed, then stir in the grated cheese and the crushed biscuits.

2. Brush a 10-inch nonstick skillet with a slightly clarified butter and place it over medium heat. Pour ½ cup of the well stirred egg combination into the pot and immediately swirl it to coat the base of the pot evenly.

3. Cook until the combination has set, about 1 ½ minutes. Using a long, wide, spatula, turn the omelet to the other side to cook for a 10-20 seconds more. Slide the omelet out onto a plate and continue making omelets in the same way until you have used all the combination. You should have about 4 omelets stacked on top of each other. Cover and keep warm.

4. Blanch, peel, core and seed all the tomatoes, placing all the seeds in a strainer set over a container. Coarsely chop 7 of the tomatoes and set them aside. Cut the remaining 4 tomatoes in half lengthwise and puree them in a blender or a food processor.

5. Press the seeds in the strainer to extract as much juice as possible. Discard the seeds and set the juice sidewise separately. In a big heavy casserole that can be took to the table, heat the olive-oil over low heat and add the onion. Cook, rousing, for about 8 minutes, or until translucent, then mixing in the garlic, paprika, cayenne pepper, bay leaf, fennel, and salt and cook for 3 minutes more, or until the garlic releases its aroma.

6. Add the exasperated carrot and the juice from the tomato, increase the heat to medium-high and cook until all of the liquid has evaporated, about 9 minutes. Add the chopped tomatoes and cook for 11 minutes, stirring occasionally, until the sauce is chunky and thick, then add the pureed tomatoes and cook just until heated through. Remove from the heat.
7. Stack 2 of the omelets, roll them up tightly, and cut crosswise into 1/4-inch-wide noodles, keeping them rolled up. Repeat with the other 2 omelets. Arrange the rolls of noodles in overlying circles on top of the tomato sauce and scatter the chopped basil over the top.
8. To serve, toss the noodles gently with the tomato sauce and Transference to individual plates.

Huevos a la Rabona

Serves: 2

Ingredients

- 4 medium eggs
- 4 bread slices
- 2 tablespoons rocoto (or any red hot chili pepper, finely diced)
- 2 tablespoons vegetable oil
- 1 tablespoon vinegar or lime juice
- 1 tablespoon oil
- ½ red onion (finely diced)
- salt and pepper to taste
- 2 tablespoons cilantro leaves, chopped (optional)

Method

1. First, put the onion and rocoto in a container, cover with cold water and rest for 10 minutes. Drain well.
2. Transference onion and rocoto mix to a container and add cilantro leaves, salt, pepper, vinegar and 1 tablespoon oil. Reserve.
3. Toast the bread in the oven or a skillet until lightly golden. Put 2 slices in each plate. (You can also fry it with some oil, which is the original way of making this dish).
4. Heat the vegetable oil in a small frying pot and fry the eggs, sunny-side-up. Season with salt.
5. Put a fried egg on top of each toast.
6. Put a tablespoon of the onion combination on top of each fried egg, and serve immediately.

Cachangas

Serves: 2

Ingredients

- 1 ½ cups flour
- 2 tablespoons salt (plus more for sprinkling, optional)
- 1 tablespoons oil + more for frying
- ¾ cup water
- ½ tablespoon baking powder

Method

1. Start by mixing all the dry ingredients in a medium container (flour, salt, baking powder if using).
2. Make a small well in the middle and add oil, mix a slightly with a fork.
3. Add water slowly – maybe add half of it and mix well. Then add a slightly bit more, until you reach the right consistency. You want the dough to be dry enough to handle, but wet enough that there is some elasticity in it. It's easier if you work the dough with your hands.
4. Form small balls (about the size of a golf ball) and set them aside. You should have about 8 – 10 balls. If less that's alright, your cachangas will be slightly bigger; if more, then your cachangas will be slightly smaller.
5. Pour some oil – enough to cover the base – on a frying pot. (The key here is to NOT BURN the oil). I can cook the cachangas on med-high (#8 on the knob/dial thing) without burning the oil, but still getting them thoroughly cooked and golden brown.
6. When the oil is nice and warm, start flattening the dough balls. You can squish them between your palms and then

carefully expotd them from the contours. If the dough rips a slightly , that's ok. It enhances character and makes that section extra crunchy. They need to be slightly thin so they can cook fast and not burn.

7. Sprinkle some salt on cachangas as they are cooking (optional)

8. Cook each side until they are golden brown. (I use a fork to go them over – occasionally spatulas just don't work)

9. Enjoy your cachangas plain, with a slightly bit of salt sprinkled on top, or with honey or maple syrup poured on.

Tropical Fruit Salad with Bee Pollen

Serves: 2

Ingredients

- 1 ripe mango (cubed)
- 1 cup papaya (cubed)
- 1 cup pineapple (cubed)
- 1 banana (sliced)
- 2 tablespoons coconut flakes
- 1 teaspoon bee pollen
- ½ orange (juiced)

Method

1. Gently combine all of the fruit in a medium container.
2. Pour the orange juice over the fruit and stir gently.
3. Sprinkle with coconut flakes and bee pollen.

Peruvian Tamales Criollos

Serves: 35

Ingredients

- 2 ½ pounds pork chops (no bones)
- 2 pounds white corn (peeled)
- 1-pound banana leaves (cut in 12-inch X 18-inch pieces)
- ½ pound fresh pork fat
- 100 grams roasted peanuts (ground)
- 100 grams black olives (preferably Peruvian)
- 50 grams sesame seeds (roasted)
- 10 ears cob corn on the (without kernels)
- 8 garlic cloves (fresh, peeled)
- 6 medium egg yolks
- 6 red chili (dried)
- 2 chilies (fresh yellow, roasted, Aji MIrasol)
- 2 hard-boiled egg (cut into eight pieces, wedges, not slices)
- 2 tablespoons vinegar
- 2 cups water
- ½ teaspoon ground pepper
- ½ teaspoon ground cumin

Method

1. The original recipe is done with Peruvian white corn, it has the biggest grain in the world and it can be cut off the cob and peeled to prepare for the recipe, but you can substitute it for just the frozen bags that you can find in any grocery store. Preferably, grind the corn using a

grinding machine, not blender (as last resource you can blend the corn in a good blender using very slightly liquid). Set aside.

2. Blend the salt, pepper, cumin, vinegar and red dried chili (previously roasted and deveined).
3. Cut the meat into medium sized pieces and marinade for about an hour in the previous mix.
4. Brown the meat in a teaspoon of lard, add the left-over marinade and the two cups of water, and bring it to a boil, simmer to cook for two hours. Remove the pieces of meat and set aside.
5. Add the broth to the corn, the rest of the lard, peanuts, sesame seeds, 6 yolks and the glass of Pisco (if you can't find Peruvian Pisco leave it like that, don't substitute).
6. Work the dough until it makes "eyes", or air bubbles. Set aside.

To put the tamales together:

1. Take about three spoonsful of dough and place them on the center of a piece of banana leaf.
2. Dig a hole in the middle and place a piece of meat, a piece of egg, an olive, one peanut, and a wedge of the fresh aji Mirasol, this may be stand in for by any fresh chile, although the aji Mirasol or aji amarillo (yellow chile) has a very distinctive flavor and is just mildly spicy.
3. Close the hole on the dough by adding a slightly bit more dough or folding and tapping it closed, pushing some of the surrounding dough on it.
4. Wrap well with the banana leaf, closing tightly all four sides on top of the dough. Use extra piece of banana leaf to covering the tamal again starting on the opposite direction and tie tightly using a string cut out of some more banana leaf or a common piece of string. Set aside.

5. Place the corn cobs at the bottom of a deep pot (rather big or medium size) and some of the banana leaves on top of the corn cobs.
6. Add just enough water to cover the leaves.
7. Place the tamales vertically and side by side so the steam travels freely through them and cover them with the rest of the banana leaves.
8. Cook for about 4 hours. Serve with onion salad called salsa criolla.

Salsa Criolla:

1. Chop a whole onion julienne style, rinse once with water and salt, and pat dry.
2. Cut one or two small tomatoes in thin wedges.
3. Add two tablespoons of mint leaves, two tablespoons of cilantro leaves, and one fresh aji amarillo (yellow chile) deveined and sliced.
4. Toss everything together and add the juice of half a lime, freshly squeezed.
5. Season with salt and pepper to taste.
6. Serve each tamal warm, unwrapped, and with a couple of spoonsful of salsa criolla on top.
7. Decorate topping with a branch of parsley or cilantro. For breakfast place a roll of fresh French bread on the side of the dish.

Chapter 4: Potini Breakfast Recipes

Apple Manchego Potini

Serves: 2

Ingredients:

- 2 soft rolls, split
- 4 tablespoons quince paste or fig jam
- Olive oil, to brush
- 1 apple, cored, sliced (peeling is optional)
- Manchego cheese slices, as required
- Salt to taste

Method:

1. Switch on the Potini press and let it preheat.
2. Brush the cut part of the rolls with olive oil. Spread with quince paste or fig jam.
3. Place apple slices on the bottom part of the rolls. Place cheese slices over the apple slices. Sprinkle with salt. Cover with the top half of the rolls.
4. Place the sandwiches in the Potini press. Operate the press following the manufacturer's instructions. Cook for 3-5 minutes depending on how crisp you like.
5. Serve right away.

Omelet

Serves: 2

Ingredients:

- 2 ounces fresh spinach
- 4 slices bacon
- 4 eggs, whisked
- Salt to taste
- Pepper to taste

Method:

1. Switch on the Potini press and let it preheat.
2. Place bacon onto the press. Operate the press following the manufacturer's instructions.
3. Cook for about 2 minutes or until crisp.
4. Remove the bacon with a slotted spoon and set aside on a plate that is lined with paper towels. Do not discard the fat remaining in the press.
5. Sprinkle half the spinach over the press. Pour half the eggs over the spinach. Sprinkle with salt and pepper.
6. Operate the press following the manufacturer's instructions and let it cook for a minute.
7. Carefully remove the omelet from the press and place on a serving plate. Serve with half the bacon.
8. Repeat the above 3 steps to make the other omelet.

Hash Browns

Serves: 2-3

Ingredients:

- 15 ounces (from a 30 ounces package) frozen, shredded potatoes
- Salt to taste
- Pepper to taste
- ¼ teaspoon paprika
- 3 tablespoons olive oil

Method:

1. Switch on the Potini press and let it preheat.
2. It is not necessary to thaw the potatoes. Add all the ingredients into a container and stir.
3. Make the hash brown in batches. Spread about 2-3 tablespoons of the combination or according to the size you desire, onto the press.
4. Operate the press following the manufacturer's instructions and let it cook for 5-10 minutes, depending on how crisp you prefer it to be.
5. Repeat with the remaining combination.

Spotish Chorizo and Pear Potini

Serves: 2

Ingredients:

- 2 soft rolls, split
- Spotish chorizo slices, as required
- 4 tablespoons fig jam
- Olive oil, to brush
- 1 pear, cored, peeled, sliced
- Manchego cheese slices, as required
- Salt to taste

Method:

1. Switch on the Potini press and let it preheat.
2. Brush the cut part of the rolls with olive oil. Spread on fig jam.
3. Place pear slices on the bottom part of the rolls. Layer with chorizo slices.
4. Place cheese slices over the chorizo slices. Sprinkle with salt. Cover with the top half of the rolls.
5. Place the sandwich in the Potini press. Operate the press following the manufacturer's instructions for 3 to 5 minutes.
6. Serve right away.

Breakfast Burritos

Serves: 3

Ingredients:

- 1 small jalapeño, deseeded, finely chopped
- 2 teaspoons fresh lime juice
- 1 large avocado, peeled, halved, pitted
- 1 ½ tablespoons olive oil + extra to brush
- ½ green bell pepper, deseeded, chopped
- ½ red bell pepper, deseeded, chopped
- Freshly ground pepper to taste
- Salt to taste
- 6 eggs
- 3 ounces cheddar cheese, grated
- 1 small clove garlic, minced
- A handful fresh cilantro, chopped
- 6 ounces Yukon gold potatoes, boiled, peeled, diced
- 3 thick cut bacon slices
- 3 large burrito style flour tortillas
- Salsa to serve
- Sour cream to serve

Method:

1. Add garlic, ¼ teaspoon salt, jalapeño and lime juice into a mortar and pestle and pound until a coarse paste is formed.
2. Transference into a container. Add avocado and mash coarsely. Add cilantro and stir.
3. Taste and adjust the salt if necessary.
4. Switch on the Potini press and let it preheat.

5. Meanwhile, place a nonstick pot over medium heat. Add 1 tablespoon of oil. When the oil is heated, add the bell peppers and sauté until tender.
6. Add potatoes and sauté until thoroughly heated.
7. Add salt and pepper and stir. Turn off the heat. Cover with a lid and set aside.
8. Place bacon on the press. Operate the press following the manufacturer's instructions.
9. Cook for about 2 minutes or until crisp.
10. Remove the bacon with a slotted spoon and set aside on a plate that is lined with paper towels. When cool enough to handle, crumble the bacon.
11. Wipe the press clean off the bacon fat.
12. Add eggs, salt and pepper into a container and whisk well.
13. Place another nonstick pot over medium heat. Add remaining oil. When the oil is heated, add egg and scramble the eggs. Cook until done.
14. Spread the tortillas on the countertop. Divide the egg among the tortillas and place at the center.
15. Sprinkle bell peppers, bacon and cheese. Wrap into a burrito. Brush the outside of the burrito with a slightly oil.
16. Cook in batches if required.
17. Operate the press following the manufacturer's instructions. Cook for 2-3 minutes or until the crispiness you desire is achieved.
18. Serve right away with salsa and sour cream.

Low Fat Vegan Silken Tofu Omelet

Serves: 1-2

Ingredients:

For omelet:

- 6-7 ounces firm or extra firm silken tofu
- 1 ½ tablespoons nutritional yeast
- ½ teaspoon Dijon mustard
- Salt to taste
- Smoked paprika to taste
- 2 tablespoons almond milk or coconut milk
- 1 ½ tablespoons cornstarch or tapioca starch
- 1/8 teaspoon turmeric powder
- Freshly ground pepper to taste

For filling:

- A handful shredded spinach
- 2-3 tablespoons sautéed onions
- 2-3 tablespoons sautéed mushrooms
- Toppings of your choice
- Vegan cheese, as required

Method:

1. Add all the ingredients of the omelet into a blender and blend until smooth.
2. Switch on the Potini press and let it preheat.
3. Pour about half the combination on the plate of the Potini press. Use lesser batter if you want a smaller omelet.

4. Operate the press following the manufacturer's instructions and let it cook for a couple of minutes or until cooked.
5. Meanwhile, warm the toppings.

6. Carefully remove the omelet from the press and place on a serving plate. Place a slightly of each of the filling ingredients over the omelet and serve.
7. Repeat the above 4 steps with the remaining combination.

Chapter 5: Norwegian Breakfast Recipes

Norwegian Thin Potcakes

Makes: 4 potcakes

Ingredients:

- 1 egg
- 1 ½ cups milk
- 10 tablespoons white flour
- 1 teaspoon granulated sugar
- 1/8 teaspoon salt
- Butter, to grease

Method:

1. Add sugar and egg into a container and beat well.
2. Add the milk and salt.
3. Add flour and mix until well combined.
4. Place a skillet over medium heat. Grease with butter.
5. Pour about 2-3 tablespoons of the combination into the pot. Swirl the pot so that the batter spreads.
6. Cook until golden brown on both sides
7. Repeat the above 3 steps to make the remaining potcakes.

Baked Cheese Omelet

Serves: 2

Ingredients:

- 2 eggs

- ¼ teaspoon salt

- 2 green onions, thinly sliced

- 1 medium bell pepper, deseeded, chopped

- 2 tablespoons water

- 1 tablespoon butter

- ½ cup cooked ham, diced

- 6 ounces Jarlsberg cheese or any other cheese of your choice, cut into ½ inch cubes

- A handful parsley, chopped, to garnish

Method:

1. Add eggs, water and salt into a container and whisk well.

2. Place an ovenproof pot over medium heat. Add butter. When butter melts, add onion, bell pepper and ham. Cook for 2-3 minutes. Turn off the heat.

3. Pour egg into the pot. Place cheese cubes on top.

4. Place the pot in a preheated oven.

5. Bake at 400°F for 15-20 minutes or until the omelet is cooked.

6. Garnish with parsley and serve.

Risengryn - Norwegian Rice Porridge

Serves: 3

Ingredients:

- 6 tablespoons short grain rice, rinsed, soaked in water for an hour

- ¾ cup water

- 2 cups milk

- ½ teaspoon ground nutmeg

- ¼ cup raisins or black current (optional)

- ½ teaspoon salt

- ½ teaspoon vanilla extract (optional)

To serve: Use as much as required

- Butter

- Sugar

- Milk

- Ground cinnamon

Method:

1. Place a saucepot over medium heat. Add water and bring to the boil.

2. Add rice and stir. Stir in the milk, vanilla and raisins if using. Bring to the boil.

3. Lower heat and cover with a lid. Simmer until rice is tender.

4. Add salt and stir.

5. Ladle into containers and top with butter, sugar, milk and cinnamon

Blueberry Breakfast Crepes

Serves: 8

Ingredients:

- 6 eggs

- 3 tablespoons butter, melted

- 2 tablespoons sugar

- 6 tablespoons butter or more if required

- Granulated sugar, as required

- Lemon wedges to serve

- 2 cups milk

- 1 ½ cups flour

- ½ teaspoon salt

- 3 cups fresh blueberries

- Powdered sugar, to taste, sifted

- Butter, melted, as required (optional), to serve

Method:

1. Add eggs to a container. Whisk well. Add about a tablespoon butter and milk and whisk well.

2. Mix together in a container, blueberries and sugar. Set aside.

3. Mix together in a container, sugar, flour and salt.

4. Add into the container of eggs and whisk well.

5. Place a shallow frying pot of about 8 inches diameter, over medium heat. Add a slightly of the butter (about ½ tablespoon).

6. When butter melts, spoon about 3 tablespoons of the batter on the pot. Swirl the pot so that the batter spreads.

7. Cook until both sides are golden brown.

8. Place a slightly of the blueberries on one half of the crepe. Fold the other half over the filling. Carefully slide the crepe on to a plate.

9. Repeat the above 4 steps with the remaining batter to make 7 more crepes.

Real Swedish Potcakes

Serves: 2

Ingredients:

- 1 egg

- 1 ¼ cups milk

- Butter, to fry, as required

- 10 tablespoons plain wheat flour

- ½ teaspoon salt

Method:

1. Add egg flour and salt into a container and stir.

2. Pour milk, a slightly at a time, and mix well each time. You will be left with a very thin batter.

3. Place a skillet over medium heat. Grease with butter.

4. Pour about 2-3 tablespoons of the batter on the pot. Swirl the pot so that the batter spreads.

5. Cook until both sides are golden brown.

6. Carefully slide on to a plate.

7. Repeat the above 3 steps to make the remaining potcakes.

8. You can stack the potcakes after it is cooked. Keep warm until use.

9. Serve with whipped cream and jam of your choice.

Swedish Scrambled Eggs

Serves: 4

Ingredients:

- 8 eggs

- 2 tablespoons fresh dill, finely chopped or 3 teaspoons dried dill

- Salt to taste

- Pepper to taste

- 8 ounces cream cheese, chopped into small cubes

- ¼ teaspoon garlic powder

- Nonstick cooking spray

Method:

1. Add eggs into a container and whisk until pale and foamy.

2. Add rest of the ingredients and stir until well combined.

3. Place a skillet over high heat. Spray cooking spray over it.

4. Add the egg combination into the pot. Lower heat to medium and stir. Scramble and cook the eggs until the consistency you desire is achieved.

Danish Kringle

Makes: 16

Ingredients:

- 2 refrigerated pie crusts, softened as per the instructions on the package
- 2/3 cup packed brown sugar
- 1 cup powdered sugar
- 4-6 teaspoons milk
- 1 1/3 cups pecans, chopped + extra to top
- 6 tablespoons butter, softened
- ½ teaspoon vanilla extract
- Water, as required

Method:

1. Place the piecrusts on a baking sheet. Do not grease the baking sheet.

2. Add pecans, butter and brown sugar in a container.

3. Divide the pecan combination among both the piecrusts and spread on half the crusts. Leave a gap of ¾ inch on the edges. Brush the edges of the piecrust with water.

4. Fold the other half over the filling. Press the edges to seal. Prick the edges as well as the top with a fork.

5. Place the kringles towards the center of the baking sheet.

6. Bake in a preheated oven at 375 °F for 15-20 minutes or until golden brown on top.

7. Cool and slice into wedges and serve.

Ableskiver – Danish Doughnuts

Serves: 5-6

Ingredients:

- 2 cups flour

- 3 teaspoons baking powder

- 4 eggs

- 2 tablespoons sugar

- A pinch salt

- 3 cups milk

Method:

1. Add flour, baking powder, sugar and salt into a container and stir.

2. Whisk together eggs and milk in a container and add into the container of flour.

3. Mix until well combined. Do not over beat.

4. Preheat an electric Ableskiver pot according to the manufacturer's instructions.

5. Pour ¼ teaspoon oil in each well. When the oil heat, pour batter into the cavities of the pot up to ¾.

6. Cook until both sides are golden brown. Remove the doughnuts and place in an oven to keep warm.

7. Top with butter and a sprinkle of sugar or a preserve of your choice.

Rugbrod - Scandinavian Rye Bread

Makes: 1 small loaf

Ingredients:

- ¼ cup rye berries, rinsed, drained

- ¼ cup millet, rinsed, drained

- 2 cups whole grain rye flour

- ½ envelope active dry yeast (about 1/8 ounce)

- ½ cup bread flour

- ½ cup + ¼ cup rolled oats

- 2 ½ cups + 2 tablespoons warm water

- 1 tablespoon fine sea salt

- Vegetable oil, to grease

Method:

1. Add rye into a small saucepot. Pour 1 cup water. Place over medium-heat and take to the boil.

2. Lower heat and simmer until dry and the rye berries are slightly tender. Transference on to a sheet of parchment paper and allow it to cool.

3. Add millets into a small saucepot. Pour ½ cup water. Place over medium-heat and take to the boil.

4. Lower heat and simmer until dry and the millets are slightly tender. Transference on to a sheet of parchment paper and allow it to cool.

5. Fit the stand mixer with the paddle. Add yeast into the container of the stand mixer. Pour remaining water. Let it sit for 10-15 minutes until frothy.

6. Add salt, rye flour and bread flour into the container. Set the mixer on low and mix for about 3-5 minutes.

7. Raise the speed to medium and mix for about 2 minutes.

8. Add millet, rye berries, and ½ cup oats. Continue mixing until well combined.

9. Place the dough into a large greased container. Cover the container cling wrap. Place it in a warm area for 2-4 hours or until it doubles in size.

10. Sprinkle remaining oats on your countertop. Place the dough on the oats and roll until the oats are coated on the dough.

11. Shape the dough into a loaf and place it in a small loaf pot. Cover the pot with a moist kitchen towel. Place in a warm area for 1 ½ - 2 hours.

12. Preheat the oven at 450° F and then bake the bread for 40-50 minutes or until light brown on top.

13. Remove the bread from the oven and place on a wire rack to cool.

14. Remove from the loaf pot and cool completely.

15. Slice and serve.

Danish Bubble

Serves: 2

Ingredients:

- 1 medium onion, finely chopped
- 1 cup leftover meat, chopped
- 1 cup cooked potatoes, cubed, cold
- 3 slices bacon, lightly cooked, chopped
- 4 tablespoons oil or butter
- 1 teaspoon Worcestershire sauce
- Salt to taste
- Pepper to taste
- 2 eggs
- 2 teaspoons butter.
- ½ cup cheddar cheese, grated
- ½ bunch chives, chopped

Method:

1. Place a skillet over medium heat. Add 1-tablespoon oil. When the oil is heated, add meat and cook until brown. Remove the meat and set aside.

2. Add 1-tablespoon oil to the skillet. Add potatoes and cook until crisp and golden brown on all the sides. Remove the potatoes and set aside.

3. Add remaining oil into the skillet. Add onions and sauté until translucent.

4. Stir in the meat, chives, bacon and potatoes. Mix well. Heat thoroughly. Sprinkle salt and pepper. Add Worcestershire sauce and stir.

5. Meanwhile, cook the eggs, sunny side up in butter.

6. Divide the bubble into 2 plates. Place egg on top. Sprinkle cheddar cheese on top and serve.

Norwegian Romme Grot

Serves: 2-3

Ingredients:

- 10 ounces sour cream

- 20 ounces whole milk

- 12 ounces all-purpose flour

- 1 teaspoon salt

- Ground cinnamon, to taste

- Salted butter, to taste

- Sugar, to taste

Method:

1. Stir constantly throughout the cooking process.

2. Add sour cream into a pot. Place the pot over low heat. When sour cream melts, sprinkle a slightly flour at a time and whisk well each time.

3. As it starts becoming thicker, add a slightly milk after each addition of flour. Whisk well each time. Continue this process until all the flour and milk is added. Do not forget to stir constantly.

4. In a while it will begin to boil. Let it simmer for a couple of minutes.

5. Add butter, sugar and cinnamon and stir. Let it simmer for 2-3 minutes.

6. Ladle into containers and serve.

Creamy Curried Egg Salad Sandwich

Serves: 4

Ingredients:

For creamy curried egg salad:

- 8 eggs, hard boiled, peeled, chopped

- 4 tablespoons mayonnaise

- 2 teaspoons curry powder

- 4 tablespoons yogurt

- Salt, as per taste

To serve:

- 8 slices rye bread

- 8 cherry tomatoes, halved

- Chopped chives to garnish

- 1 cup alfalfa sprouts

Method:

1. To make creamy curry salad: Add mayonnaise, curry powder, yogurt and salt into a container and stir well.

2. Add eggs and fold gently.

3. Toast the bread slices.

4. Take 8 slices of bread and place on a serving platter. Divide the egg combination over the bread. Spread it evenly over it. Sprinkle alfalfa sprouts over it. Sprinkle chives. Place tomatoes on top and serve right away.

Scandinavian Breakfast Muesli

Serves: 2

Ingredients:

For muesli:

6. 1 cup rolled oats

7. 2 teaspoons quinoa flakes

8. 4 tablespoons nuts of your choice, chopped

9. 2 teaspoons flaxseeds

10. 4 tablespoons unsweetened coconut flakes

11. 4 tablespoons dried berries

To serve:

- Milk or yogurt

- Maple syrup

Method:

1. Add all the ingredients of muesli into a container and toss.

2. Transference into an airtight container and place in a dry area.

3. To serve: Take the required amount of muesli in a container. Add milk or yogurt. Drizzle maple syrup on top and serve.

Ollebrod - Danish Rye Bread Porridge

Serves: 6

Ingredients:

- 1/3 cup malt syrup

- ¾ pound stale rye bread, cut into 1 inch cubes

- 1 ½ teaspoons vanilla extract

- 3 tablespoons unsalted butter

- 6 tablespoons heavy cream to serve (optional)

- 1 cup apple juice

- 12 ounces dark, malty beer

- 2 strips orange peel

- 1 ½ teaspoons ground cinnamon

- ¾ teaspoon ground cardamom

- ¼ teaspoon kosher salt or to taste

- Fresh fruits of your choice to serve (optional)

Method:

1. Place rye bread in a container. Pour beer over it. Cover and place it at room temperature overnight.

2. Add the bread combination into a saucepot. Pour ¾ cup water, apple juice, malt syrup and vanilla and stir. Also add orange peel, cinnamon and cardamom and stir.

3. Place the saucepot over medium high heat.

4. When it begins to boil, lower heat and simmer for 6-7 minutes until thick. Stir occasionally. Mash the bread cubes with the back of your ladle or spoon.

5. Turn off the heat. Discard orange peels. Add butter and salt and stirring up until butter melts.

6. Ladle into containers. Place a blob of cream.

7. Serve with fruits if using.

Chapter 6: Nigerian Breakfast Recipes

Moi Moi (Beans Cake)

Servings: 4

Ingredients:

- 500g beans/black eyed peas
- 7 small chili pepper
- 4 fresh tomatoes
- 4 boiled eggs (optional)
- 2 ½ cooking spoons of palm oil or vegetable oil
- ½ clove garlic or ginger
- leaves, sandwich bags or aluminum cups
- cooked fish/sardines
- salt and pepper to taste
- 60g shrimps (optional)

Method:

1. First, soak the Beans/Black eyed peas for not longer than 30 – 45 minutes, wash and peel off the brown back of the beans by rubbing the beans with your palms until it becomes white then wash carefully. Be sure to remove all the brown peels.
2. Wash the beans till all is clean white, add onions, red chili pepper, tomatoes, chopped small garlic and a bit of ginger (very slightly), blend all together.
3. Boil the eggs, shrimps and fish.
4. Add 2 tablespoon of vegetable oil and seasoning like Maggi/salt then stir, taste if seasoning is okay.
5. Slice the egg and shred the fish make sure to take away the bones.

6. Rinse the leave/sandwich bag/aluminum cups, fold into a cone brake the bottom backward to avoid leakage, pour the grounded beans, add few shrimps, fresh sliced eggs and wrap the leave.
7. Put water in a cooking pot and add all the wraps inside cover to cook for 30mins.
8. Open one covering to see if cooked and solid.

Plantain Mosa (Plantain Potcake)

Servings: 6 medium potcakes

Ingredients:

- 3 tablespoons plain flour (all-purpose flour)
- 2 tablespoons evaporated milk (peak milk)
- 1 overripe plantain
- 1 large egg or 2 medium eggs
- ½ teaspoon salt
- ground cayenne pepper (to taste)
- cool water
- vegetable oil (for frying)

Method:

1. First, break the egg into a container, beat and set aside.
2. Peel the overripe plantain and mash with a fork till a good blend is achieved.
3. Add cool water to the solid plantain bit by bit and mix on each occasion till you get a medium reliability.
4. Pass the medium consistency blend through a sieve into the egg. Mix very well.
5. Sift the plain flour into the combination from Step 4. Mix thoroughly.
6. Add salt, cayenne pepper and evaporated milk and stir very well. It is ready to be fried.
7. Set your frying pot over medium heat and pour a small quantity of vegetable oil; just enough to grease the frying pot. This should be about 1 tablespoon of oil.

8. When hot, pour a small amount of batter into the pot to make a 5mm thick and 5-inch diameter plan-cake.
9. Keep an eye on it and once you see the edge of the plan-cake caking, flip it to fry the other side too.
10. It is ready when both sides are light brown.
11. Fry the rest of the dough using steps 8 to 10.

Nigerian Fried Plantains and Eggs

Servings: 1-2

Ingredients:

- 2 ripe plantains
- 2 large eggs or 3 medium eggs
- 1 fresh tomato
- pepper to taste
- a small onion bulb
- seasoning (as you prefer)
- salt to taste
- vegetable oil for frying

Method:

1. First, cut off the top and bottom of the plantain. Make a low cut on the side and peel of the skin from that point.
2. Next, cut the plantains to any figure of choice. You can sprinkle some salt on the plantain if you like salted plantains.
3. Temperature up the oil and fry the plantains until brown.
4. Now chop the onions, tomato and pepper.
5. Break the eggs, add salt to taste and whisk until double in size.
6. Heat up a slightly oil on the pot; add the tomato, onions and pepper; stir fry for some seconds and add any seasoning of choice.
7. Next, add the creamed eggs and leave to cook for some seconds. Then turn it over, so that the another side will cook as well.

8. Now the eggs are ready to be served with the cooked plantains.

Akara (Nigerian Bean Cakes)

Serves: 2-4

Ingredients:

- 2 habanero peppers (also chili peppers)
- 1 cup of beans (black-eyed or brown beans)
- 1 medium onion
- salt to taste
- vegetable oil for frying

Tools you will need:

- blender
- mortar and pestle

Before you fry akara:

- Remove the beans coat. It is important that you do not let salt come in interaction with the beans you will use in making Akara till you are ready to fry it. Salt is believed to destroy the leavening property of beans. This is what stops spattering of the beans batter during frying.
- Soak the beans in water for 3 hours to make it soft enough for your blender. If you will grind it using the durable grinders in Nigerian markets, it will not be necessary to soak the beans for extended periods of time.
- Cut the pepper and onions into necessary sizes.

Method:

1. First, grind the beans with your blender making sure you add as slightly water as possible. The water should be just enough to move the edges of your mixer. Do not add any another ingredient when grinding the beans. It is supposed that other ingredients, if added too early, reduce the ability of the ground beans particles to stick composed.

2. Set some coconut oil on the cooker to heat up. The oil should be at least 3 inches deep.

3. Put some of the ground beans into a mortar. This should be the amount you can fry in one go.

4. Stir the beans puree with the pestle in a nonstop circular motion. You need to apply some weight so that you can energize the particles of the beans puree.

5. This stirring technique releases the gas that will act like a leavening agent to the bean's particles, making them rise and somehow stick together. This will be like the yeast making the dough rise in Puff Puff or what foldaway does to cake batter.

6. Keep stirring till the ground beans appears whiter and you can perceive its peculiar aroma.

7. Add some water till you get the consistency shown in the video below.

8. Check to make sure the oil is hot. The oil should be hot enough to sizzle but not too hot. If too hot, the Akara will splash as soon as the beans batter hits the oil.

9. Once the oil is hot, add the onions and pepper to the beans puree in the mortar. Stir well.

10. Add salt to your taste and stir again. Salt should always be added just before scooping the beans combination into the oil. If salt stays in the combination for extended

periods of time, it will destroy the leavening property of the beans. This stuff is what makes the Akara float in the oil and prevent spatter during frying.

11. To fry the Akara, scoop the combination with a table spoon and slowly pour this into the oil. Dipping the spoon a slightly bit into the oil helps reduce spatter.
12. Fry the bottom till brown and flip to fry the top side too.
13. When the Akara balls are brown all over, remove and place in a mesh lined with paper towels.

Nigerian Chicken Shawarma

Servings: 6-8

Ingredients:

- 2 chicken breasts(de-boned/boneless)
- 2 chicken thighs (de-boned/boneless), you can also use de-boned/boneless beef
- 7+ shawarma bread (either pita bread/flour tortilla censorships)
- 4 medium sized carrots
- 2 big tomatoes (cut into thin strips)
- 2 small sized cabbage
- 2 large cucumber (cut into thin strips rings)
- 2 medium sized onion
- 1 tablespoon olive oil (for stir frying)
- ketchup
- mayonnaise

For the marinade:

- 2 teaspoon curry
- 1 teaspoon thyme
- 1 tablespoon vegetable /olive oil
- 1 teaspoon onion powder/2 teaspoons minced onions
- 1 teaspoon garlic powder/2 teaspoons minced garlic
- 1 large chicken stock cube/bouillon cube (crushed into dust)
- half a teaspoon black pepper

- chili pepper to taste
- salt to taste (optional)

Method:

1. Start by washing and cutting the vegetables into thin strip (if you haven't done that yet) and set aside. Also Cut the chicken or beef into thin carpets and set aside. *Tip: I recommend using a combination of chicken thighs & breasts, because the fat from the thighs adds extra flavor and compliments the taste of the chicken breast.*

2. Place the chicken strips into a container, add the marinade and mix thoroughly until well incorporated. Then cover and store in the fridge for 3 to 25 hours. Tip: You don't have to wait 24 hours, you can just store it overnight or for 2-3 hours, but I realized that the longer the meat marinades, the better it tastes.

3. In a pot, heat up a tablespoonful of oil. Add the steeped chicken/beef & stir fry until juicy and brown. Scoop unto a plate and set aside.

4. Mix some mayonnaise and ketchup together.

5. Place a shawarma bread on a clean flat surface and cut into two equal sizes (that's if you are using a large pita bread).

6. But if using a very flat bread or tortilla wraps, simply, spread the" mayo-ketch" on it and then fill it with the sliced vegetables on one end and sprinkle some chili pepper (optional).

7. Then fold the bread, tuck in the edge, and roll to form a shawarma wrap

Nigerian-Style Potato and Egg

Servings: 4

Ingredients:

- 5 lb. (2.2 kg) yukon gold potato (1 bag, boiled)
- 7 oz (200 g) chopped tomato
- 7 oz (200 g) baked beans (in tomato sauce)
- 4 oz (115 g) sardines
- 6 medium eggs or 5 large eggs (beaten)
- 4 tablespoons butter (cut into small pats)
- 3 tablespoons canola oil
- 1 medium onion (sliced into rings)
- 1 teaspoon garlic (minced)
- 1 teaspoon pepper
- 1 teaspoon salt
- 1 teaspoon red chili flakes

Method:

1. First, heat the oil in a medium nonstick pot over medium heat.
2. Add the onion, garlic, pepper, salt, and chili flakes, and cook for a 1-2 minutes, but don't let the onions brown.
3. Add the tomatoes, sardines, and baked beans, and cook for 4-5 minutes until the liquid reduces a bit.
4. Stir in the eggs and cook for about 2-3 minutes. Remove the pot from the heat.
5. Place a pat of butter on 3-4 potatoes, then spoon the egg combination on top.
6. Serve hot.

Yamarita (Nigerian Egg Battered Yam Fries)

Serves: 1-2

Ingredients:

- 1-pound puna yam
- 2 large egg or 3 medium eggs
- ¾ cup all-purpose flour
- ¼ garlic powder
- ¼ curry powder
- ¼ black pepper
- ¼ thyme
- ¼ salt
- cayenne/chili pepper to your taste
- salt
- water
- a slightly powdered bouillon (optional)

Method:

1. Start by peeling the yam and cut into rectangles about 1 inch wide and 1/2-inch-thick and rinse and drain.
2. Put the yams inside a pot, add water about the level of the yam, also add a ½ teaspoon of salt and let it cook for about 7 minutes.
3. Drain off the excess water and Transference the yam to a container of cold water to stop the cooking process.
4. Once the yams are cooled drain off the water and set aside.

5. Crack the eggs in a container, add a pinch of salt and cayenne pepper to your taste and whisk together also set that aside.
6. In a separate container add the flour, garlic powder, curry powder, thyme, black pepper and bouillon and mix together.
7. Now deep the yam (one at a time if possible) in the egg and flour combination respectively making sure the yam is well coated.
8. Heat up the oil and fry the yam turning halfway between until golden brown.
9. Serve with your favorite sauce or eat as is.

Nigerian Coconut Bread

Servings: 8

Ingredients:

- 3 ½ cups flour (plus more for kneading)
- 3 tablespoons butter or 3 tablespoons non-hydrogenated vegetable shortening (melted)
- 2 tablespoons sugar
- 1 (¼ ounce) package active dry yeast
- 1 cup coconut milk
- ¾ teaspoon salt
- ½ cup unsweetened coconut (finely grated)
- ½ cup warm water

Method:

1. First, put coconut, sugar, yeast and water into a small non-reactive container and stir briefly.
2. Set aside until combination is swollen and bubbly, about 15 minutes.
3. Mix flour and salt together in a large container.
4. Add yeast combination, coconut milk and butter; using your hands or a wooden spoon, stir until well combined.
5. Turn dough out onto a well-floured surface and knead, dusting with more flour as necessary, until soft and elastic, 5 to 6 minutes.
6. Form dough into a ball, dust generously all over with flour and Transference to a clean large container.

7. Cover container with a kitchen towel and set aside in a warm spot to let rise until doubled in size, about 1 ½ hours.
8. Divide dough into 8 pieces and roll each into a ball.
9. Arrange balls of dough on a large greased baking sheet, spacing them 3 to 4 inches apart.
10. Set aside in a warm spot, uncovered, to let rise until doubled in size again, about 45 minutes.
11. Preheat oven to 350°F.
12. Bake bread until deep golden brown and cooked through, 20 to 25 minutes.
13. Serve warm or set aside to let cool to room temperature.

Nigerian-Style Club Sandwich

Servings: 4

Ingredients:

- 16 slices thin white sandwich bread (crusts cut off)
- 8 slices chicken breast
- 4 canned sardine fillets
- 4 tablespoons unsalted butter (softened)
- 2 hard-boiled eggs (peeled and sliced)
- 1 small carrot (finely shredded)
- ½ plum tomato (cored, seeded and finely hacked)
- ¼ cup mayonnaise
- ¼ head green cabbage (finely shredded)
- salt and pepper

Method:

1. Mash the sardines in a small container with a fork.
2. Add the softened butter and mash together until smooth and well combined. Set aside.
3. Stir together the shredded cabbage, carrot, tomato, and mayonnaise in a container until well combined. Season to taste with salt and pepper.

To assemble:

1. Lay a piece of bread on your work surface.
2. Spread a thin layer of sardine butter over the bread, then top with 1 slice of chicken breast.
3. Top with another piece of bread, and spread some of the cabbage slaw over it.

4. Arrange a few slices of hard-boiled egg over the slaw, then top with a third slice of bread.
5. Lay 1 slice of chicken breast over the bread.
6. Spread a thin layer of sardine butter over a fourth slice of bread and lay it over the chicken, buttered-side down.
7. Repeat with the remaining ingredients to make 3 more sandwiches.
8. Cut each sandwich in half and serve.

Eggless Nigerian Potcakes

Servings: 3

Ingredients:

- 2 tablespoons butter
- 1 cup milk
- 1 or 1 cup mashed/pureed ripe banana
- ½ cup premium whole wheat flour
- ½ cup white all-purpose flour
- ¼ cup sugar
- ¼ teaspoon ground pepper
- ¼ teaspoon salt
- ¼ teaspoon nutmeg
- vegetable oil or cooking spray (for frying)

Method:

1. First, take a tablespoon of oil and add to your pot on medium heat. Spread the oil over the pot evenly. The oil is mostly to prevent sticking, so you need very slightly oil.
2. Once the oil is hot, use a ½ cup or any other cup you wish to pour in the potcake mix. Tilt the pot all around to spread the mix evenly.

3. Once the potcake starts cooking and coming together and you can gently get a fish slice all the way under the potcake, turn it over.

4. Keep flipping till both sides are well done. Keep the heat on low-medium heat to prevent the potcakes from burning/browning too much.

5. Repeat steps 1-4.

Nigerian Egg Stew

Servings: 5

Ingredients:

- 8 large eggs or 9 medium eggs (beaten)
- 3 tablespoons tomato paste (watered down with ½ cup of water)
- 1 habanero or scotch bonnet pepper
- 1 cup cooking oil
- 1 large onion (chopped)
- 1 stalk of spring onions (for garnishing)
- ½ green bell pepper (chopped)
- ½ red bell pepper (chopped)
- ½ tablespoon garlic (crushed)
- salt/ bouillon cube (to your taste)

Method:

1. First, heat up oil, add onions and garlic. Sauté onions and garlic till onions softens.
2. Pour in tomato paste. Fry tomato paste for about 3 mins while stirring to prevent burning.
3. Add in the chopped red and green bell peppers. Cook for another 2 minutes on low heat and it's ready to get in your belly. After cooling down to warm though.

4. Add the cup of water to the beaten eggs then gradually stir the egg/water mix into the bubbling stew. Stir continuously to break up the eggs.

5. Serve with boiled or fried plantains, boiled or fried yams, boiled or fried potatoes or a mix all three.

Nigerian Bread and Egg Casserole

Servings: 2-4

Ingredients:

- 7 large eggs or 8 medium eggs (beaten)
- 3 to 4 slices of bread
- 3 red bell pepper
- 2 stock cubes
- 1 tablespoon butter
- 1 green bell pepper
- medium sized onion
- salt to taste

Method:

1. First, chop the peppers, tomatoes, onion, and garlic. Grease an eight-inch dish with some butter and set aside
2. Sauté peppers and onions with butter for about 5 minutes. Sauté peppers and onions
3. Add the garlic, then tomatoes and the rest of the spices. Let it cook for another 3 minutes. (I added a slightly ugu leaves, this is totally optional). Add tomatoes and garlic
4. Tear the bread in small pieces into the casserole dish.
5. Pour in the cooked vegetables, add the eggs. Mix till ingredients are well incorporated.
6. Bake in the oven for about 20- 30 minutes.
7. Serve hot and enjoy.

Nigerian Potato Hash

Servings: 1-2

Ingredients:

- 4 medium sized red bell pepper
- 3 to 4 cloves of garlic
- 3 large potatoes
- 2 tablespoons butter
- 1 medium sized onion
- ½ teaspoon each of curry powder, ginger powder, and dried thyme leaves
- minced meat (the quantity depends on how much of it you want in your potato hash)
- salt to taste

Method:

1. First, peel and wash potatoes. Chop into bite size pieces. Also chop the peppers, onions and garlic.
2. Put the potato in a pot with cold water, add some salt, and boil for about ten minutes (don't overcook, just allow to boil till it becomes soft and the color starts to change). Drain out the water, and set aside.
3. Melt butter and sauté the peppers with onions. After about five minutes add the garlic, and all the other spices

(it is best to add the garlic after the peppers have cooked a bit, so it doesn't overcook and taste bitter).

4. Add boiled minced meat, stir together and add the potatoes. Let it cook for another ten minutes, or till the potatoes are well cooked.

5. Serve with fried egg and fresh juice. Enjoy.

Nigerian Sausage, Peppers, and Onions Bake

Servings: 1-2

Ingredients:

- 1 medium size red and green bell pepper
- sausage (whatever you like)
- onions
- salt to taste

Method:

1. Wash peppers, and take out the seeds. Peel back of onions and wash. Now chop them and put into a baking pot.
2. Add salt to the vegetables, put in the oven and let it bake for about 10 minutes.
3. Slice sausages and add to the vegetables (my vegetables were already half way cooked, if yours is raw, you may want to mix it with the vegetables at the very beginning so that everything cooks together).
4. Let it bake for another 10 minutes, be careful not to overcook the vegetables.
5. Serve hot and enjoy.

Ewa Agoyin (Boiled Beans with Pepper Sauce)

Serves: 1-2

Ingredients:

- 2 cigar cups (approx. 500g) brown/black eyed beans
- 5 cooking spoons red palm oil
- 5 big plum tomatoes
- 2 stock cubes
- 1 handful crayfish
- 1 big onion
- salt and pepper to taste

Before you cook ewa agoyin:

- Soak the beans in cold water for 5 hours. Boil the beans for 5 minutes and discard the water. Rinse the beans in cold water and set aside. This soaking and pre-cooking process will help reduce the gas inducing elements.
- Chop the onions, grind the crayfish and pound the pepper.
- Blend the tomatoes and boil the tomato puree till all the water has dried from it.
- Pre-cook the diced onions without any added water. The aim is to get it to caramelize a bit so that it will take less time to fully caramelize during frying.

Method:

1. First, cook the beans till done. For ewa agoyin, the beans need to be very soft. *(Note: if you have a pressure cooker, it is one of the staple foods you will want to use it for. It considerably reduces the cooking time.)*

2. When the beans are done, add salt, leave to dry up all the water and set aside.

3. To cook the agoyin, pour the palm oil into a separate dry pot. Allow to heat up till the oil starts smoking and the red color changes to clear. It is well to do this at medium heat so that the oil does not get too hot too quickly.

4. To keep the smoke to a minimum and still have the traditional taste of ewa agoyin, use vegetable oil and when it is very hot, add a small amount of palm oil.

5. Now add the precooked onions and stir continuously till the onions is fully caramelized. It should be very dark in color.

6. Add the parboiled tomato puree and stir continuously till you cannot tell the difference between the tomatoes and onions.

7. Add the pepper, crayfish, stock cubes and salt to taste. You can also add a slightly water at this point if you want.

8. Stir very well and bring to the boil.

9. Serve by dishing the beans into a plate and scoop some agoyin stew on it. Ewa agoyin can be eaten on its individual, with soft and stretchy bread (known as ewa ati bread) or with fried plantains.

Bread Boat

Servings: 2-3

Ingredients:

- 5-10 baby spinach leaves
- 4 medium eggs or 3 large eggs
- 1 cooking spoon olive oil
- 1 small red onion
- 1 tablespoon diced sweet peppers (fresh paprika)
- 1 bar of baguette
- ¼ ground black pepper
- salt (to taste)

Method:

1. First, beat the eggs.
2. Add the salt, black pepper, onions and spinach. Stir very well.
3. Pour the olive oil in a frying pot and when it heats up, pour in the egg mix and spread it out.
4. After about 20 seconds, stir the egg gently. Keep stiring from time to time till the egg cakes all over. You want bold scrambled eggs.
5. Cut a long baguette bread into two.
6. Make a hole in each one like you are making a boat.
7. Fill up the hole with the scrambled eggs.
8. Serve on its own with chilled fruit juice or hot chocolate.

Chapter 7: Muffin Tin Breakfast Recipes

Bacon-Wrapped Eggs

Servings: 6 cups

Ingredients:

- 12 bacon strips
- 6 medium-large eggs
- chives (chopped)
- salt
- black pepper

Method:

1. Start by heating the oven to 400° F. Prepare a baking sheet by cover it with aluminum foil.
2. Put bacon on the baking sheet and bake until half-cooked. Let cool until the bacon can be handled.
3. Prepare muffin tin by spraying the cups with non-stick spray or greasing it with butter.
4. Line muffin tin cups with bacon, using 2 strips per cup. Repeat until you have 6 bacon cups.
5. Add an egg into all of the bacon cups. Sprinkle salt, pepper, and chives to taste.
6. Bake the cups for 10 to 12 minutes, or until the egg whites have hardened, but the yolks are still runny. The bacon should be crispy but not burned.
7. Carefully scoop the bacon cups out of the muffin tin and serve while still hot.

Poached Eggs

Servings: 4 eggs

Ingredients:

- 4 medium-large eggs
- 4 slices of whole-wheat toast (for serving)
- chopped parsley (for serving)
- water
- salt and pepper to taste

Method:

1. Start by heating the oven to 350° F.
2. Pour a tablespoon of water into each muffin tin cups.
3. Put an egg over each muffin cups. Be careful so the yolks don't break. Season with sprinkles of salt and pepper.
4. Bake to desired doneness, around 8-15 minutes.
5. Take out of the oven and carefully scoop eggs out with a spoon.
6. Serve with a sprinkle of chopped parsley on top and toasts on the side.

Buttermilk Potcake Muffins

Servings: 8 muffins

Ingredients:

- 4 tablespoons sugar
- 1 ½ cups buttermilk
- 1 ½ tablespoon canola oil
- 1 medium-large egg
- 1 cup all-purpose flour
- 1 teaspoon baking powder
- 1 teaspoon baking soda
- 1 teaspoon salt

Method:

1. Start by heating the oven to 350° F. Grease 8 muffin tin cups using butter or non-stick spray.
2. Whisk together flour, sugar, salt, baking soda, and baking powder in a large container until well combined. Add in egg, buttermilk, and oil. The batter's consistency should be thick with small lumps. Don't over-mix the batter.
3. Fill about 1/3 of each muffin tin cups with the batter. Bake in the oven for 12-15 minutes, until the muffins are cooked thoroughly.
4. Loosen up muffin edges using a small spatula and scoop it out.
5. Serve with whipped cream, syrup, or any other toppings of your choice.

Veggie Frittata Cups

Servings: 12 frittatas

Ingredients:

- 8 medium-large eggs
- 2 handfuls of spinach (roughly chopped)
- 1 cup cherry tomatoes (halved)
- 1 cup mushrooms (sliced)
- ¾ cup cheddar cheese (grated)
- ½ cup milk
- ½ teaspoon salt
- ½ teaspoon pepper
- fresh rosemary, parsley, and basil to taste

Method:

1. Start by heating the oven to 350° F. Lightly coat 12 muffin tin cups with non-stick spray to prevent sticking.
2. Put in eggs, milk, cheese, salt, and pepper in a large container, stir until well-combined. Add in cherry tomatoes, mushrooms, and spinach.
3. Scoop the egg combination into the molds. Add some more cheese on top. Sprinkle rosemary, parsley, and basil.
4. Bake in the oven for about 18-22 minutes. Check periodically after the 15 minutes mark so they don't get burned. Pierce the center of the frittata with a knife to check if they're done (a clean knife means they are cooked through).

5. Let cool for 5-10 minutes. Glide a butter knife to loosen up the edges and take the mini frittatas out.
6. Serve and enjoy.

Frozen Yogurt Bites

Servings: 12 cups

Ingredients:

- 2 tablespoons honey
- 1 cup blackberries
- 1 cup Greek yogurt
- ¼ cup milk

Method:

1. Mix together the Greek yogurt, milk, and honey in a medium-large container. The consistency should be thick and pourable.
2. Place paper or foil cupcake liners inside 12 muffin tin cups. Divide yogurt combination evenly among the cups. Sprinkle the blackberries on top of each cup.
3. Freeze the yogurt bites for at least 2 hours or until firm. Remove cup liners before serving.

Peanut Butter Cereal Cups

Servings: 12 cups

Ingredients:

For the beans and soffritto:

- 4 cups cereal of your choice
- 2 tablespoons butter
- ½ cup honey or maple syrup
- ½ cup peanut butter

For the plantains:

- 1 ½ tablespoons yogurt
- ¼ cup white chocolate chips

Method:

Make the frosting:

1. Put the white chocolate chips and yogurt in a small microwaveable cup. Heat in the microwave until they're melted. Stir so the combination is smooth. Set aside.

Make the cups:

1. Melt butter in a big pot over medium heat. Add the honey and peanut butter. Stir until well mixed. Add in cereal. Toss until the cereal is well-coated.
2. Grease muffin tin cups using non-stick spray. Press the cereal combination into the cups firmly, so they're well-packed.
3. Allow to cool completely for 12-15 minutes or place them in the refrigerator for about 8-10 minutes.

4. Remove cereal cups from the tin. Drizzle white chocolate frosting on top of the cups.
5. Serve and enjoy.

Parmesan Hash Brown Cups

Servings: 6 cups

Ingredients:

- 2 medium-large potatoes (peeled)
- 2 tablespoons olive oil
- ½ teaspoon salt
- ½ teaspoon black pepper
- 1/3 cup parmesan cheese (grated)
- ¼ cup potko breadcrumbs
- ¼ teaspoon garlic powder (optional)

Method:

1. Start by preheating the oven to 350° F. Use non-stick cooking spray to grease the muffin tin.
2. Grate the potatoes by hand using the coarsest blade of a box grater. Every once in a while, place potatoes inside triple layered paper towels and wring out over the sink. The drier they are, the crispier the hash browns will be.
3. Insert grated potatoes, parmesan cheese, potko breadcrumbs, and olive oil into a large container. Season with salt, black pepper, and garlic powder. Stir until well-combined.
4. Scoop potato combination into muffin tin cups. Bake until the hash browns are golden with brown edges, or for about 40 minutes. Start checking your hash browns at the 30-minute mark to avoid burning. Note that baking can take more or less time, depending on the potatoes you are using and their moisture level.

5. Take you the muffin tin and allow to cool on a rack for 10-15 minutes. Gently run a butter knife along the cup rims to take out the hash browns.
6. Serve with sour cream, ketchup, or any other condiments of your preference.

Granola Containers with Strawberry Yogurt

Servings: 12 medium containers

Ingredients:

For granola cups:

- 1 ¼ cups quick-cook rolled oats
- 1 medium-large egg
- 1 teaspoon lemon zest
- ¾ teaspoon cinnamon
- ½ cup raisins
- ½ cup dried apricots (chopped)
- ½ teaspoon salt
- ½ cup honey
- ½ cup chopped almonds
- 1/3 cup wheat germ
- 1/3 cup chia seeds
- ¼ teaspoon allspice
- ¼ cup coconut oil (melted)

For strawberry yogurt:

- 2 ½ tablespoons strawberry jam
- 1 ½ tablespoons sugar
- 1 cup plain yogurt
- ¼ cup strawberries (diced)

Method:

To make the yogurt:

1. Combine yogurt and strawberry jam in a mixing container. Mix well. Adjust the sweetness by adding

155

sugar. Add in diced strawberries and stir to combine. Chill in the refrigerator.

To make the granola cups:

1. Start by preheating the oven to 350° F.
2. Mix oats, wheat germ, chia seeds, raisins, almonds, cinnamon, apricots, lemon zest, allspice, and salt in a large container.
3. Using another container, whisk egg, honey, and oil. Pour wet ingredients to the dry combination gradually. Stir until the combination is well-mixed.
4. Grease the muffin cups with non-stick spray or coconut oil. Wet your fingers and start dividing the granola combination among 12 medium-sized muffin cups. Form granola containers with your fingers, starting from the middle and working your way up to the edges.
5. Bake for 20 minutes, or until the edges turn brown. Let sit to cool for 5-10 minutes, then take the containers out of the molds.
6. Add a small scoop of strawberry yogurt on top of the granola containers before serving. Serve immediately so the containers don't become soggy.

Baked Oatmeal

Servings: 12 medium cups

Ingredients:

- 2 medium-large eggs
- 1 ½ cups 2% milk
- 1 cup steel-cut oats (not instant)
- ½ cup dried cranberries
- ½ cup walnut pieces
- ½ cup pumpkin seeds
- ½ teaspoon cinnamon
- ½ teaspoon nutmeg
- ¼ teaspoon salt
- ¼ cups natural peanut butter
- maple syrup (for serving)

Method:

1. First, soak oats with water and refrigerate overnight to soften.
2. Heat the oven to 400° F.
3. Drain oats. Mix oats with dried cranberries, walnuts, pumpkin seeds, cinnamon, nutmeg, and salt. In another container, whisk eggs and add in with milk and peanut butter. Add dry elements to wet and stir to syndicate.
4. Divide and place oat combination into 12 medium-sized muffin cups. Bake for 20 minutes until cooked thoroughly. Test if the oats are done by inserting a toothpick (the toothpick will come out dry and clean if they're done).
5. Let cool for about 5-10 minutes. Take oat cups out of their molds.

6. Drizzle with maple syrup and serve.

Chapter 8: Moroccan Breakfast Recipes

Khobz (Moroccan Bread)

Servings: 2 loaves

Ingredients:

- 4 cups flour (high-gluten or bread flour preferred)
- 2 teaspoons salt
- 2 teaspoons sugar
- 2 tablespoons vegetable oil
- 1 ¼ cups warm water
- 1 tablespoon yeast (active dry)

Method:

1. First, prepare two baking sheets by lightly oiling them or by dusting the pots with a slightly cornmeal or semolina.
2. Mix the flour, salt, and sugar in a large container. Make a large well in the center of the flour combination and add the yeast.
3. Add the oil and the water to the well, stirring with your fingers to dissolve the yeast first, and then stirring the entire contents of the container to incorporate the water into the flour.
4. Turn the dough out onto a floured surface and begin kneading the dough, or use a stand mixer fitted with a dough hook. If essential, add flour or water in very small amounts to make the dough lenient and pliable, but not sticky. Continue kneading for 10 minutes by hand (or 5 minutes by machine), or until the dough is very smooth and elastic.
5. Divide the dough in half and shape each portion into a smooth circular mound. (If you prefer, you can divide the

dough into four to six smaller loaves instead.) Place the dough onto the prepared pots, cover with a towel and allow it to rest for 10 to 15 minutes.

6. After the dough has rested, use the palm of your hand to flatten the dough into circles about ¼-inch thick. Cover with a towel and let rise about 1 hour (longer in a cold room), or until the dough springs back when pressed lightly with a finger.

7. Heat an oven to 435 F/225 C.

8. Create steam vents by scoring the top of the bread with a very sharp knife or by poking the dough with a fork in several places. Bake the bread for about 20 minutes—rotating the pots about halfway through the baking pots—or until the loaves are nicely colored and sound hollow when tapped. Transference the bread to a rack or towel-lined basket to cool.

Harcha (Moroccan Semolina Pot-Fried Flatbread)

Serves: 6-8

Ingredients:

- 3 tablespoons sugar
- 3 cups (400 grams) fine semolina
- 2 teaspoons baking powder
- ½ to ¾ cup (120 to 180 milliliters) milk
- ½ cup (125 grams) soft or melted butter
- ¼ teaspoon salt
- ¼ cup coarse semolina (optional)

Method:

1. First, blend together the fine semolina, sugar, baking powder, and salt in a mixing container. Add the butter, and blend with your hands or a wooden spoon just until the combination is the consistency of sand and the semolina grains have all been moistened.
2. Add ½ cup milk and mix until dough forms. It should be quite moist, wet nearly, and easily packed into a big mound. Add additional milk if necessary, to achieve this consistency.
3. Shape the dough into balls any size that you like and leave the dough to rest a few minutes.
4. Preheat a griddle or frying pot over medium-low heat. While the griddle is heating, roll the balls in the coarse semolina (if using) and flatten each ball into a disc about ¼-inch thick, or a bit thicker if you like.

5. Cook the harcha over fairly low heat, about 5 to 10 minutes on each side, until they turn a pale to medium golden color. Flip only once, and check rarely to be sure the harcha aren't coloring too quickly, as they need some time to cook all the way through.
6. Serve immediately with jam, cheese, or butter.

Krachel (Moroccan Sweet Rolls with Anise and Sesame)

Servings: 12-15

Ingredients:

- 4 ½ cups flour
- 2 teaspoons anise seeds
- 2 medium-large eggs (lightly beaten)
- 2 tablespoons orange flower water
- 1 tablespoon yeast
- 1 ½ teaspoons salt
- ¾ cup warm milk
- ½ cup sugar
- ½ cup butter (melted or very soft)
- egg wash made from 2 egg crushed with 2 tablespoon milk
- 1 tablespoon golden sesame seeds (for sprinkling on the rolls)

Method:

1. Start by dissolving the yeast in a few tablespoons of warm water and set aside.
2. Combine the flour, sugar, salt and anise seeds in a large mixing container. Add the eggs, the butter, the oil, the orange flower water, the yeast, and the milk. Mix to form a very soft, sticky dough.
3. If you find the dough is too sticky to handle, add the smallest amount of flour necessary to be able to knead the dough. If the dough lacks tackiness, work in extra warm milk or water a few tablespoons at a time.

4. Knead the dough on a lightly floured surface (or in a stand mixer with a dough hook) for about 10 minutes, or until very smooth. (For the desirable light-textured rolls, it's necessary to have the dough somewhat sticky; you'll find that it becomes much easier to handle after its first rising.)
5. Transference the dough to an oiled container and turn the dough over once to coat it with oil. Cover the container with a towel and leave the dough to rise until doubled – Usually, this takes about one to one-and-a-half hours, but leave the dough to rise longer if necessary.
6. After the dough has risen, punch it down, gather it up and turn it over. Cover with the towel and leave for a second rising for about an hour (longer in cool weather), until light and spongy.
7. Turn the dough out onto your work surface and divide it into 12 to 15 smooth, evenly shaped balls. Place the balls of dough two inches apart on an oiled baking sheet (or a pot lined with parchment paper).
8. Allow the dough to rest a few minutes, then flatten the balls of dough. Refuge the baking sheet with a towel and leave the dough to rise another hour or longer, or until the rolls are very light and puffy.
9. Preheat an oven to 450 F (230 C). Brush the tops and margins of the rolls with the egg wash and sprinkle the rolls with sesame seeds.
10. Bake the krachel for 15 to 20 minutes, or until rich golden brown. Transference the rolls to a rack to cool.

Khlea and Egg

Serves: 2-4

Ingredients:

- 4 heaped tablespoons khlea
- 6 medium-large eggs
- pinch of salt
- pinch of cumin
- freshly ground black pepper
- a very small amount of fresh parsley (finely chopped)
- 1 tablespoon double (heavy) cream (optional)

Method:

1. Beat the eggs lightly with a fork, with the pinch of salt.
2. Heat the tagine on medium high heat over a diffuser.
3. Add your cold khlea to the cool tagine and wait for the tagine to heat up and the fat to melt. This might take up to 10 minutes. Give it a stir every now and then.
4. When the fat has melted, scoop some out, I usually get rid of about 1 - 2 tablespoons, depending on how much fat was clinging to the meat. Do not increase the fat back to your cold khlea in the jar. If you like, you can use it in another bowl but in the attention of food safety, do it within the next two of hours.
5. Stir the khlea a slightly and let it warm up for about 30 seconds.
6. Pour the beaten egg into the tagine. Now it's not going to sizzle up like it would if you're using a frying pot.

7. Let it settle for about 20 - 30 seconds, then stir it, breaking it up, like you would, when making scrambled eggs. Continue responsibility this for about 6 minutes, let it set, stir, set and stir. You'll only need to do this about 3 - 4 times.

8. When the eggs look like they are losing most of their liquid, drizzle in the cream, if using. Stir once more if the egg isn't too set. If you can't stir, just consent the cream to be absorbed.

9. When the egg tagine looks like it's almost cooked, take it off the heat, sprinkle the cumin, pepper and chopped parsley all over and serve immediately, with any type of bread you fancy.

Shakshouka (Moroccan Eggs Tagine)

Yield: 2-3

Ingredients:

- 4-6 free-range eggs
- 3 tablespoons olive oil
- 2-3 button mushrooms (sliced)
- 2 rashers of bacon (diced into cubes)
- 1 ½ cups diced tomatoes (tinned or fresh)
- 1 red or brown onion (roughly diced)
- 1 medium red pepper (capsicum/bell pepper), sliced or diced
- 1 garlic clove (chopped)
- ½ long red chili (finely diced)
- ½ teaspoon salt
- ½ teaspoon ground cumin
- ½ teaspoon paprika
- ½ teaspoon ground coriander seed powder
- ½ dried or fresh oregano leaves (parsley or thyme can be used instead)
- ½ teaspoon turmeric powder (optional) – alternatively, use 1+ 1/2 teaspoons of pre-mixed moroccan spice mix
- fresh parsley and/or coriander (cilantro), roughly chopped

Method:

1. First, heat a teaspoon of olive oil over medium-high heat in a deep-frying pot and add the bacon. Cook until crispy,

then remove to a container but reserve the fat in the frying pot.

2. Add the remaining olive oil. Add the onions, chili and peppers and sauté for 3-4 minutes, until slightly softened. Season with salt and add the mushrooms and garlic. Cook for a minute, stirring.

3. Then add back the bacon and spices, stir for 30 seconds allowing the aromas to be released. Add the tomatoes, stir and cover with the lid. Cook on medium-low temperature for 11-13 minutes, giving it a stir a few times.

4. Using a spoon, make small wells in the tomato mix and crack an egg into each, letting the egg whites to spill over the edges. Sprinkle each egg yolk with a slightly salt and pepper, cover with a lid and cook on medium-low heat until the egg whites settle and firm up but the egg yolks remain gooey, about 5 minutes. It's very easy to overcook the eggs this way, so it's best to leave them slightly under-cooked as they will keep cooking while getting served.

5. Serve the eggs in the cooking dish sprinkled with some fresh parsley and coriander.

Moroccan Omelet

Serves: 1

Ingredients:

- 9 grape tomatoes
- 1 teaspoon fresh lemon juice
- 1 small clove garlic (minced)
- 1 medium-large egg plus 3 large egg whites (beaten)
- ¾ cup baby spinach
- ½ cup canned chickpeas (rinsed and drained)
- ¼ small red onion, diced (about ¼ cup)
- ¼ cup low-sodium vegetable broth
- ¼ avocado (sliced)
- 1/8 teaspoon ground cumin
- pinch each ground coriander, turmeric, cinnamon and black pepper

Method:

1. Cook onion in broth in a nonstick skillet over low heat until translucent, about 6 minutes.
2. Add tomatoes, lemon juice, garlic, spices and chickpeas; cook, stir-ring irregularly, until tomatoes have cooked down somewhat, 4 to 5 minutes. Transference to a pot.
3. Wipe skillet and mist with vegetable oil spray. Pour in eggs, then spinach; cook up until eggs set, 5 minutes.
4. Fold omelet; plate, top with chickpea mix and enhancer with avocado.

Moroccan Sausage and Egg Tagine

Serves: 4

Ingredients:

- 8 oz./225 g. merguez (or other sausage)
- 6 medium-large eggs
- 2 medium tomatoes (peeled, seeded and chopped)
- 1 medium-large onion (finely chopped)
- ½ teaspoon salt
- ½ teaspoon cumin
- ¼ teaspoon black pepper (or 1/8 teaspoon cayenne pepper)
- handful of olives (green pitted, sliced)
- small handful of chopped cilantros (or parsley)
- salt to taste
- cumin to taste
- chopped cilantro (or parsley), garnish

Method:

1. First, gather the ingredients.
2. Cook the sausage in a large skillet or in the base of a tagine until the meat tests done. If there is a big amount of fat from the sausage, remove the extra, leaving enough to stay cooking. If the sausage was low-fat, you may need to add a slightly olive oil to the pot at this point.
3. Add the onion, tomatoes, olives and seasoning and cook for about 5 minutes. Pour the eggs nonstop over the sausage and vegans. Break the yolks, and allow the eggs to simmer until set.

4. To help this along, you can lift the edges of the eggs as they cook and tip the pot to allow uncooked egg to run underneath and cook faster. If cookery the eggs in a tagine, cover the eggs and agree them to poach until done.

5. Dust the top of the cooked eggs with cumin and salt to taste, garnish with a slightly chopped parsley, and serve.

Baghrir (Moroccan Potcakes)

Servings: 8

Ingredients:

- 2 ½ cups warm water
- 1 cup farina flour
- ½ tablespoon dry yeast
- ½ cup all-purpose flour
- ½ tablespoon baking powder
- a dash of salt, about 1/8th teaspoon

Method:

1. Start by combining water, yeast, flour, semolina and salt in your blender, pulse until everything mixes well together.
2. Add the Baking powder and mix again.
3. Place in a container and cover to rise, will take approximately 30 minutes.
4. After 30 minutes, the batter should be thin and not thick as the usual potcakes. *
5. Heat an 7" skillet over average heat, pour about 1/2 cup of the batter into the skillet. Batter should spread to the edges of the skillet, if not then thin it with more water. see notes for clarification.
6. Small holes should appear all over the surface, continue cooking until no obvious uncooked surface appears. Took me 3 minutes to be totally cooked. **
7. Let them cool down a bit before serving.
8. Serving suggestions: Traditionally, these are enjoyed with butter and honey. Also, for a salty twist, sometimes

can be trundled over olive oil and hard-boiled eggs (cut into small pieces. Practically, this can be enjoyed with your favorite syrup.

Msemen (Square Laminated Potcakes)

Servings: 20

Ingredients:

- 3 ½ cups white flour, all purpose or bread
- 2 teaspoon sugar
- 2 teaspoon salt
- 1 ½ cups warm water (not hot)
- ½ cup fine semolina or durum flour
- ¼ teaspoon dry yeast (less in very warm weather)

For folding the msemen:

- 1 cup vegetable oil (more if needed)
- 1 cup fine semolina
- ¼ cup very soft unsalted butter (more if needed)

Method:

Make the msemen dough:

7. First, mix the dry ingredients in a large container. Add the water and combine to make a dough.
8. Knead the dough by hand (or with a mixer and dough hook) until very smooth, soft and elastic but not sticky. Adjust water or flour as necessary to achieve that texture.
9. Divide the dough into balls the size of small plums. Be sure the top and sides of the balls are smooth. Transference the balls of dough on an oiled tray, cover loosely with plastic and leave to rest for 10 to 15 minutes.
10. While the dough is resting, set up a work area. You'll need a large flat surface for spreading and folding the dough.

Set out containers of vegetable oil, semolina and very soft butter.

11. Set your griddle or large frying pot on the stove, ready to heat up.

Shape the msemen:

1. Generously oil your work surface and your hands. Dip a ball of dough in the oil and place it in the center of your work space.
2. Using a light touch and quick sweeping motion from the center outward, gently spread the dough into a paper-thin, roughly shaped circle. Oil your hands as often as required so that they slide easily over the dough.
3. Dot the flattened dough with butter and sprinkle with semolina. Fold the dough into thirds like a letter to form an elongated rectangle. Dot over with butter, sprinkle with semolina, and fold again into thirds to form a rectangular.
4. Transference the folded dough to the oiled tray and repeat with the remaining balls of dough. Keep track of the order in which you folded the squares.

Cooking the msemen:

1. Heat your griddle or frying pot over medium heat until quite hot. Initial with the first msemen you folded, take a square of dosh and place on your oiled work surface. Oil your hands and pat the dough resolutely to flatten it to double its original size.
2. Transference the flattened square to the hot griddle and cook, turning several times, until cooked through, crispy

on the exterior and golden in color. Transference to a rack.

3. Repeat with the remaining squares, working with them in the order in which they were folded. You can flatten and cook several at a time if your pot or griddle can accommodate them.

4. When each msemen has cooled for a minute or two, pick it up from opposite ends and gently flex it for a few seconds with a quick back and forth, see-saw motion. This helps separate the laminated layers from each other.

5. Serve the msemen immediately, or allow to cool completely before freezing.

Reheating and serving msemen:

1. Msemen can be reheated directly from the freezer in a frying pot placed over medium-low heat, or directly on the rack in a preheated 350° F (180° C) oven.

2. To make the traditional Moroccan syrup for dipping, heat equal portions of unsalted butter and honey in a frying pot. When hot and just beginning to bubble, turn off the heat. Dip the warm msemen into the syrup to coat the potcake on both sides.

Mlaouis

Serves: 8-10

Ingredients:

Main dough:

- 350 g of strong white bread flour
- 260-290 ml of water (lukewarm)
- 150 g of fine semolina flour
- 1 ½ teaspoon of salt
- ½ teaspoon of dried instant yeast (1 ½ teaspoon for mlaoui mkhamrine)

For shaping and laminating:

- 200 g of fine semolina flour
- 110 g of butter
- 100 ml of vegetable oil

Method:

Prepare the dough:

1. First, mix the yeast with a few tablespoons of barely warm water in a small glass. Stir.
2. Place the flours, salt and yeast in a container (each in one side). Add the water to ¾ and start mixing either by hand or by machine.
3. The dough needs to be thoroughly kneaded to become smooth and soft without being sticky. It takes about 22 minutes by fingers and 12 minutes with a KitchenAid.

4. The achieve the desired dough texture, gradually add the other ¼ of water according to the absorption of the flours used.
5. You could leave the dough, covered, to rest for 15 min (in cold weather) or skip this step if the weather is too warm. For Mlaouis Mkhamrine, let the dough rise for 40-60 min at normal temperature.

Shape Mlaouis the easy method:

1. Oil your hands as well as the dough. Depending how big or small you want the Mlaouis to be. Form slightly thick sausages and roll them. Their length will define the width of Mlaouis. At all times, you should keep the dough as well as the hands oiled.
2. Place each dough sausage on a generously oiled surface. We regularly use a big tray where we place them all. Roll the bread balls in oil and cover with foil. Set aside to rest for 10 min. Usually, by the time you're done with the whole dough, you could go back to the first one you shaped and start shaping a Meloui.
3. Oil the worktop, try to flatten the dough and stretch it in length at the same time. In this way, your dough does not have to be thin to a see-through condition.
4. You could also start the Meloui shaping the same way we start Msemmen shaping by folding the outer two thirds of a see-through layer of dough on the middle third.
5. Smear with butter and sprinkle with fine semolina flour. Avoid tearing the dough.
6. Now, hold one end of dough with one hand and roll it from the other end with the other while stretching. Keep rolling tight while leaving the edges neat. It should look like this (see pictures below).
7. Tuck the ends inside and set aside for 10 min.

Second method for shaping Mlaoui:

1. Literally start the same way we do for Msemmen. Once the two thirds of the tinny dough layer are folder on the middle one without getting to the square shape. Smear the dough with butter and sprinkle it with fine semolina flour in length. Fold the dough again (3rd picture top right).
2. Stretch the dough in length again. Again, a tiny bit of butter and a sprinkle of semolina flour.
3. Shaping Mlaouis second method. 3 rolls in the middle of Msemmen waiting to be compressed to round-shaped Mlaouis
4. Like the previous method, hold one end of dough with one hand and roll it from the other end with the other while stretching. Keep rolling tight while leaving the edges neat.

Flatten Mlaoui rolls:

1. Flatten the first roll you made to 2 mm thick round Meloui.
2. Set aside while you carry on with the break of the dough rolls. This allows them to proof a bit (16-20 min).
3. Pot-fry each one on medium-heat for 3 mins or so.
4. Plain and khlii-filled Mlaouis being pot-fried.
5. Serve warm with a good glass of hot tea.
6. Freeze extra Mlaouis once cooled.

Batbout (Moroccan Pita Bread)

Servings: 20

Ingredients:

- 3 cups white flour (preferably bread flour or high-gluten)
- 3 tablespoons olive oil or vegetable oil
- 2 tablespoons sugar
- 2 cups durum flour or fine semolina
- 2 teaspoons salt
- 2 cups warm water (approx.)
- 1 tablespoon dry yeast
- 1 cup whole wheat flour

Method:

1. Start by mixing the yeast with a teaspoon of the sugar in a slightly warm water; set aside until foamy.
2. Combine the flours, remaining sugar and salt. Add the oil, water and the yeast combination.
3. Stir to bring the dough together, then knead by hand on a floured surface, or with a mixer and dough hook, until smooth and supple, but not sticky. Add flour or water in small increments as needed to make a soft, manageable dough.
4. Shape portions of the dough into smooth balls about the size of plums. Arrange the balls on a lightly floured surface with at least an inch between balls. Cover with a towel and leave the dough to rest for 10 to 15 minutes.
5. When the dough has rested, dust your work surface with flour or fine semolina and roll each ball out into a thin

round about 1/8" (0.3 cm) thick. Place on a fiber sheet or towel and cover. Leave to rise for an hour or a slightly longer, until light and puffy.

6. Heat a large pot or griddle over medium heat for several minutes until very hot. Carefully Transference the bat bout in batches to the pot. Gently turn the bat bout as soon as set (after about 12 to 17 seconds) before air bubble being to appear on the surface.

7. Continue cooking the batbout, turning gently several more times, until they have puffed with air and are browned on both sides.

8. Transference the cooked batbout to a rack or towel-lined basket to cool. Store completely cooled batbout in the freezer.

Sfenj (Moroccan Donuts)

Servings: 14

Ingredients:

- 500 gr plain flour
- 240ml lukewarm water
- 1 teaspoon salt
- 1 tablespoon dry active yeast
- ¼ teaspoon caster sugar to activate the yeast
- vegetable oil (for frying)
- 250 gr icing sugar sifted for the glaze (optional)
- 2 tablespoon milk for the glaze (optional)

Method:

1. First, activate the dry yeast by adding ¼ teaspoon of sugar and a tablespoon of lukewarm water in a small container. Stir with a fork and consent for 6 to 11 minutes until foamy.
2. Transference the flour, the salt and the water in a large container and combine all the ingredients. You should obtain a very sticky dough. If the cash is not sticky (almost like a batter consistency but thicker), add a few tablespoons of water until you obtain the right consistency.
3. Flour a worktop and knead the dough for 10 minutes until very elastic. It will be a bit challenging in the beginning as the dough is very sticky but it will get easier after a couple of minutes.

4. Transference the dough back in the container and cover with cling film and let the dough rest for 4 hours in a warm place, until the dough triples in size.
5. When ready to deep fry the donuts, heat up 6 cm (2.5 inches) of frying oil in a deep pot over medium high-heat until it reaches 180 C (350 F).
6. Dip your hands in water (to help handling the dough) and pull off a piece of dough the size of a plum. Make a hole in the center of the dough and stretch it to make a wide ring. Quickly and carefully Transference the ring of dough into the warm frying oil.
7. Fry on both sides turning occasionally, until crisp and golden.
8. Once ready, use a slotted spoon to Transference the donut to a wire rack lined with paper towels.
9. Continue frying the donuts until you've used all the dough. Enjoy very warm with everything yummy such as sugar, honey, or icing sugar glaze.
10. To make the icing sugar glaze, Transference the sifted icing sugar and milk into a medium sized container and slowly stir until smooth.

Classic Harira (Moroccan Tomato, Lentil, and Chickpea Soup)

Servings: 6-8

Ingredients:

- ½ pound meat (lamb, beef or chicken; uncooked, chopped into ½-inch pieces)
- 3 tablespoons vegetable oil
- 4 tablespoons tomato paste
- 3 cups water
- 2 to 3 tablespoons dried lentils
- several soup bones (optional)

For the stock:

- 6 medium-large tomatoes (about 2 pounds; peeled, seeded and pureed)
- 1 or 2 stalk celery (with leaves; finely sliced)
- 1 ½ teaspoons pepper
- 1 teaspoon ground cinnamon
- 1 tablespoon ground ginger
- 1 tablespoon kosher salt
- 1 bunch cilantro (finely chopped to yield about ¼ cup)
- 1 bunch fresh parsley (finely chopped to yield about ¼ cup)
- 1 large onion (grated)
- 1 handful of dried chickpeas
- ½ teaspoon turmeric (or ¼ teaspoon yellow colorant)
- smen (optional)

- 2 to 3 tablespoons rice (uncooked; or uncooked broken vermicelli, optional)

Method:

Before you begin cooking the soup:

6. First, gather the ingredients.
7. Wash the herbs and drain well.
8. Pick the parsley and cilantro leaves from their stems. Slight pieces of stem are all right, but remove long, thick pieces through no leaves.
9. Finely chop them by hand or with a food processor.
10. Soak and skin the chickpeas. (You might need to soak them the night before you cook.)
11. Peel, seed and puree the tomatoes in a blender or food processor. Or, stew the tomatoes and pass them through a food mill to remove the pits and skin.
12. Pick through the lentils and wash them.
13. Assemble the remaining ingredients and follow the steps below.

Brown the meat:

1. Put the meat, soup bones and oil into a 6-quart or larger pressure cooker.
2. Over medium heat, cook the meat for a few minutes, stirring to brown all sides.
3. Make the Stock
4. Add the cilantro, parsley, celery, onion, chickpeas, smen (if using), spices and tomatoes. Stir in 3 cups of water.
5. Cover tightly, and heat over high heat until pressure is achieved. Reduce the heat to average, and cook for 25 to 30 minutes. Take away from the heat and release the pressure.

Make the soup:

1. Add the lentils, tomato paste combination, and 2 quarts of water to the stock.
2. Set aside (but don't add yet) either the rice or vermicelli.
3. Cover the pot and heat the soup over high heat until pressure is achieved. Reduce the heat to medium and continue cooking.
4. **If adding rice:** Cook the soup on pressure for 30 minutes. Release the pressure, and add the rice. Cover, and cook with weight for an additional 20 minutes.
5. **If adding vermicelli:** Cook the soup on pressure for 45 minutes. Release the pressure, and add the vermicelli. Simmer the soup, exposed, for 8 to 10 minutes or until the vermicelli is plump and cooked.

Thicken the soup:

1. While the soup is cooking, make a (soup thickener) by mixing together the 1 cup of flour with 2 cups of water. Set the combination aside, and stir or whisk it occasionally.
2. The flour will eventually blend with the water. If the combination is not smooth when you're ready to use it, pass it through a sieve to remove lumps.
3. Once the rice (or vermicelli) has cooked, taste the soup for seasoning. Add salt or pepper if desired.
4. Bring the soup to a full simmer. Slowly — and in a thin stream — pour in the flour combination. Stir continually and keep the soup simmering so the flour doesn't stick to the bottom.
5. You will notice the soup beginning to thicken when you've used approximately half the flour combination.

The thickness of harira is up to you. Some like to thicken the broth so that it accomplishes a cream-like consistency.

6. Simmer the thickened soup, stirring occasionally, for 5 to 10 minutes to cook off the taste of the flour. Take away the soup from the heat and serve with some parsley.

Hssoua Belboula (Moroccan Barley Soup with Milk)

Servings: 6

Ingredients:

- 8 ½ cups water
- 5 to 6 oz evaporated milk
- 3 tablespoons olive oil
- 2 teaspoon cumin
- 2 cups whole milk
- 2 tablespoons butter (unsalted)
- 1 ½ cups barley grits (medium caliber)
- 1 tablespoon salt
- pepper to taste

Method:

1. First, pick through the barley to remove any debris. Wash the barley grits several times in a large container filled with water, draining each time through a sieve. Wash until the water is no longer cloudy.
2. In a small stock pot mix the barley grits, water, olive oil, salt, pepper and cumin.
3. Bring to a simmer and cook over medium-low heat for 30 to 40 minutes, or until the soup is thick like porridge and the grains are tender.
4. Stir several times during cooking, and be careful that the heat is not too high or the soup can boil over.

5. Stir in the milk and bring to a simmer again for a few minutes. Turn off the heat, and stir in the butter and disappeared milk.
6. Taste and adjust seasoning as desired. If you like, garnish each serving with a slightly cumin and olive oil or a bit of butter.

Bissara (Split Peas and Fava Beans Soup/Dip)

Serves: 4

Ingredients:

1. 400 gr dried split peas or fava beans (or a mix of both), soaked overnight
2. 4 garlic cloves
3. 3 tablespoons olive oil (and more for garnish)
4. 2 teaspoons baking soda
5. 1 teaspoon paprika (and more for garnish)
6. 1 teaspoon ground cumin (and more for garnish)
7. 3 tablespoons fresh onions (chopped, for garnish, if desired)
8. salt to taste

Method:

1. Start by draining the peas and/or fava beans, run them through water and drain them again.
2. Transference the peas and/or fava beans in a large casserole and cover with 1 liter of water (the peas and/or fava beans should be completely covered with water). Add the garlic cloves (unpeeled) and the baking soda.
3. Bring to a boil, cover with a lid and reduce the heat to low. Leave to simmer gently for 20 minutes.
4. Remove the garlic cloves from the casserole, unpeel and mash them. Transference the mashed garlic, olive oil, paprika, cumin and salt in the casserole.
5. Cover with a lid and leave to simmer for another 20 minutes to allow the peas and/or fava beans to cook and soften. Stir occasionally. If you notice that at this stage

the combination is too dry, add a few tablespoons of water.

6. Once the peas and/or fava beans combination is completely cooked and soft, run the combination through a food processor (or pass the combination through a sieve) to obtain a smooth result.

7. Serve hot with bread in a shallow dish or a container with a generous coating of olive oil, a sprinkle of paprika and cumin and some chopped onions if desired.

Loubia (Moroccan Stewed White Beans)

Servings: 6

Ingredients:

- 1 lb. dry white haricot (navy) or Cannellini beans, soaked overnight then drained
- 5 cloves of garlic (finely chopped or pressed)
- 3 tablespoons fresh parsley (chopped)
- 3 tablespoons fresh cilantro (chopped)
- 3 ripe tomatoes (grated)
- 2 teaspoons ginger
- 1 medium onion (grated)
- 1 tablespoon salt
- 1 tablespoon paprika
- 1 tablespoon cumin
- ½ cup olive oil
- ¼ teaspoon turmeric (optional)
- ¼ teaspoon cayenne pepper or fresh chili peppers, to taste (optional)
- 2 lb. beef or lamb, on the maxilla;

Method:

Optional step if using fresh meat:

1. If preparing the white beans with lamb or beef, start by browning the meat in the olive oil over medium heat. (Dried or preserved meat needs no browning.) Then proceed with one of the cooking methods below.

Pressure cooker method:

1. Place all ingredients in a pressure cooker and stir to combine.
2. Add 2 quarts (about 2 liters) of water and bring the liquids to a boil over high heat.
3. Cover, bring to pressure, then reduce heat to medium. Continue cooking with pressure for 40 minutes, or until the beans are tender.
4. If the beans are still fully submerged in sauce, reduce the liquids by simmering uncovered until the sauce is thick and not watery, but still quite ample.
5. Taste and adjust seasoning, if needed. Serve warm.

Conventional pot method:

1. Mix all ingredients in a large, heavy-bottomed pot. Add 2 quarts of water (about 2 liters) and bring to a rapid simmer.
2. Cover and continue simmering the beans over medium heat for about 1 1/2 hours, or until the beans are cooked to desired tenderness and the sauce is thick and no longer watery.
3. During cooking, stir occasionally and add a slightly water if the liquids reduce before the beans have fully cooked.
4. Taste and adjust the seasoning. Serve warm.

Conclusion

We have come to the end of the book. Thank you for reading and congratulations for reading until the end. I hope you found the book informative and interesting.

This breakfast recipe book is definitely one of the most loved, delicious, rich and healthy cook book from across the world.

The recipes often call for fresh herbs, vegetables and fruit. However, these can be replaced with frozen and canned foods as well. It is also possible to change and replace certain ingredients if you don't like them or if they are not available. You can take a judgment call on the same and replace certain ingredients to improve the texture or flavor of the dish.

Modify and experiment with these recipes and create your very own personalized recipes. Do not let cooking become a chore. Rather, make it a fun activity. The recipes in this book are easy to make and delicious. All the recipes have been tested and tasted so the end result will leave you satisfied.

Finally, if you enjoyed this book then I'd like to ask you for a favor. Will you be kind enough to leave a review for this book on Amazon? It would be greatly appreciated!

Thank you and good luck!

Made in the USA
San Bernardino, CA
09 March 2020

65484900R00111